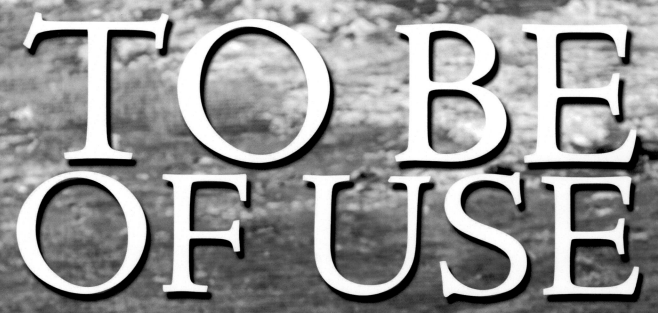

TO BE OF USE

FIVE DECADES AS A CANCER DOCTOR INCLUDING THE STORY OF THE CONQUEST OF CHILDHOOD LEUKEMIA

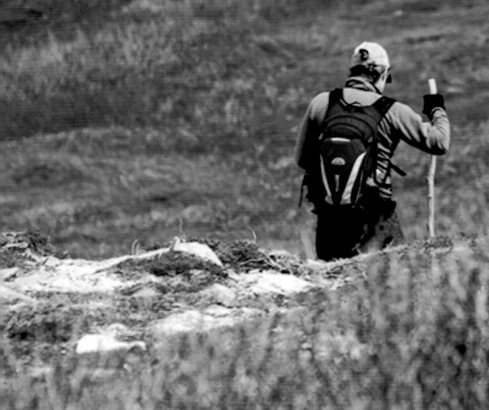

EDWARD ARENSON MD CWSP

To order additional copies of this book, contact:
Xlibris
844-714-8691
www.Xlibris.com
Orders@Xlibris.com

ISBN: 978-1-7960-9907-2 (sc)
ISBN: 978-1-7960-9906-5 (e)

Print information available on the last page

Rev. date: 08/25/2020

TO BE OF USE

FIVE DECADES AS A
CANCER DOCTOR

INCLUDING THE STORY
OF THE CONQUEST

OF CHILDHOOD LEUKEMIA

Edward Arenson MD CWSP

TABLE OF CONTENTS

Dedications

This memoir is dedicated to all of my patients without whom I would not have been taught the lessons that I have learned and without whom this book would not have been possible.

I also dedicate this book to Dr. Wilbur Larch of the Cider House Rules by John Irving.

I wish to thank my wife, Aura, and two of my daughters, Jennifer and Patty, for their help with and support of this joyful project. I also thank Aura for courageously helping me sustain my practice, despite the fatigue of advancing age, long enough to make sure that my patients were well situated to transfer and continue their care. The pain of this process was lessoned immeasurably by Aura's hard work and commitment to the task.

Finally, I would like to thank my dear friend and accomplished high school classmate, Kathleen Fulton, for her generous editorial assistance.

PREFACE

Be kind and be courageous --- Anne Frank

In these many pages, I hope to provide an account of my fifty years as a cancer and blood doctor during which I was fortunate enough to witness first hand the dramatic events and heroic people who led us out of the darkness of nearly universal death from cancer to the light of curability. My own role was limited, but I believe that my experiential insights are unique and informative. This journey is presented chronologically, for the most part, but digresses occasionally into discussions which transcend the time line of the book. When I finally reach the present, I intend to use the preceding insights and lessons to pontificate briefly on where we might have lost our way, and how we might return to the right path (*T'shuva*, Hebrew, to return to the right path).

I have written another lengthy saga, that of my alter life as a birder and naturalist. I believe that the two histories compliment each other, so chapter 22 of this book will be the same as chapter 42 of the sister book, entitled "Feathers in the Wind", Above Average Adventures of a Below Average Birder".

Your Author

CHAPTER 1

In Which I Relate My Formative Days Before I Had a Clue

I am born inauspiciously at the Philadelphia Lying-In Hospital on April 11, 1945. FDR dies the next day. Both of my parents are patients there at the same time—my mother, who is in labor, and my father, who is a Naval officer suffering from alcohol poisoning after overzealously celebrating the departure of a hated superior. I am a sickly baby, very small, about five pounds, a poor feeder and grower, and inexplicably fearful and vigilant. Several years later, Eleanor Roosevelt, FDR's widow, visits Toledo, Ohio where I live and where my mother is photographed with her and friends at a Zionist event. I don't know it at the time, but Mrs. Roosevelt would later be a model for the many high-achieving women with whom I share my profession and my life.

I contract whooping cough and pneumonia in infancy and require hospitalization. I am still haunted by my recollections of a dark, multi-bed ward where I hunker in a crib listening to conspiratorially whispering nurses, alone in the night waiting to be stuck or injected, a wakeful nightmare. The daily injections of penicillin, a new drug, probably save my life and foreshadow similar transformative events which I will experience later in my medical career. Whether I would have suffered these traumatic experiences so early in life if my parents had not filled my air with cigarette smoke, I can only guess, but I have never fully forgiven them. As a young child, I am predictably asthmatic which hampers my ability to excel athletically as all "popular" students must do. Later in life, free of smoke, I run marathons to compensate.

Thus, doctors play a major role in my early life, and, for the most part, are a positive role model. These are the days of house calls in which the good pediatrician, I.H. Cass MD, parks his black Buick in the driveway, walks with purpose to the front door, climbs the stairs, and works his magic. I always get better.

Later, an allergist, Dr. Friedmar, also a nice fellow, but a bit over-excitable, has to chase me around his office before I submit to allergy testing which requires multiple cuts in my arms with a paring knife into which he puts drops of serum to be observed for swelling and itchy reactions indicative of allergy and, of course, the need for allergy shots. Doc Friedmar and I eventually settle our differences, and, at age 8 years, I take the bus on my own to his office every week to get my shot. I had lost my fear of shots, but never lose my dread of the rickety old elevator in the medical office building. Someone in Toledo had died in an elevator plunge, and my parents, as is their Jewish obligation, make sure that I know about it.

In spite of my respiratory fragility, which persists to the present, my parents choose the saxophone to be my instrument of choice for my musical education. I learn to play it well, win awards, play in a rock-and-roll band, but sometimes cannot play when I am having an asthma attack. I "coulda been" a great drummer and have become a decent one while the saxophone sleeps silently in its case. Perhaps it will re-enter my life once I am retired if my lungs hold up.

And so, my life begins with doctors and hospitals and physical ailments with which to cope. Perhaps this sets the stage subliminally for an inclination to enter the field of medicine in which I would be in control, (if there is such a thing in life,) and might be empathetic and useful. I learn to deal with discomfort and only ask to be taken to the emergency room for shots of adrenaline when I can simply no longer breathe without them; I dislike being perceived as weak and unhealthy more than I dislike the discomfort.

These early challenges, in retrospect, plant the seeds for my future as a cancer doctor, brain tumor doctor, wound care specialist, and specialist in hyperbaric oxygen medicine. I cannot say that these early experiences produce courage, but I never seek to avoid situations where courage might be needed and, perhaps, eventually does develop. The C word, Courage, will be capitalized throughout the remainder of this narrative to emphasize its importance in the messages I wish to convey. Keeping the C word in mind, let us move on to the next step in my pathway toward medicine, my early education.

CHAPTER 2

My Scholarly Journey from English Major and Art History Minor to Medicine and a Brief Dalliance with Architecture

As a successful student at Ottawa Hills High School, an excellent suburban public school outside Toledo, Ohio, which is currently ranked number one in Ohio and in the top ten nationally, I knew I wanted to go to the best college I could as did many of my classmates. It was a very competitive academic environment which trumped other activities of early life. My parents had both attended Cornell University in the early 1940s; I wanted to go there and ultimately did.

My senior class of about 98 students distinguished itself academically more than athletically. At the time, this was a negative. Those of us who were the scholars and non- athletes, were judged unfavorably as "nerds", "bookworms", you get my meaning. From this small group of students, many of whom (about 30) had shared our education from kindergarten through high school, we sent two to Cornell U., (including myself,) one to Princeton, two to Smith College, one to Wellesley, one to Radcliffe, (our valedictorian Carol Rapaport,) one to MIT, one to Sarah Lawrence College, one to Duke U., (Susan Moore, of blessed memory, salutatorian and my girlfriend at the time, but never again,) and one to Columbia U., Mark Singer, one of my best friends, senior class president, and the only other graduate to become a physician. He became Head of the Department of Head and Neck Surgery at University of California San Francisco (UCSF).

Before leaving high school for college, I must devote a few words to two teachers that had a major impact on my future. I would guess that nearly all successful people can attribute some of their success to one or two outstanding teachers. These will be the first of a short list of people who appear in this book and whom I will categorize and recognize as *menches*, the Yiddish word for righteous people of strength and honor. As it turns out, there are eighteen of these special people. For those that are interested in numbers, eighteen is the number in the Jewish heritage that means chai, or life, and from which the expression *l'chayim*!, to life!, is derived.

Mensch 1: Ethel B. Sager, my Latin teacher for four years, ninth through twelfth grade, was a prototypical "spinster" teacher who devoted herself to her profession. She was not only an excellent and inspirational Latin teacher, but a scholar who took interest in "her" promising students. She might forgive a late paper as long as the result was worth the wait. She never raised her voice and didn't need to. The most memorable advice she gave me and others, which I have never forgotten and have passed on to my own students and children, was "seek to know something about everything and everything about something". I believe that I have actually come close to achieving this challenging goal, and for that I am ever grateful to Miss Sager.

Mensch 2: Mrs. Helen Braun was my eighth grade English teacher. She was a German lady who placed high value on precision and discipline. She had an abiding concern for the survival of a "civilized society" in which people had respect for one another and demonstrated this daily by adhering to standards of manners and speaking correctly. It was not possible to get through a school year with Mrs. Braun successfully without understanding the fundamentals of grammar, at the "Strunk and White" level, and knowing the codes of contemporary manners that she taught. Once these manners were understood well enough to satisfy this teacher, it was likely that they would be observed in real life experiences. That has been the case with me, for the most part, and the grammar was not a means unto itself, but a metaphor for doing things the right way. She, like Miss Sager, undoubtedly has affected my deportment nearly every day of my life. Again, I have only gratitude for the challenges they gave us.

Edward Arenson MD CWSP

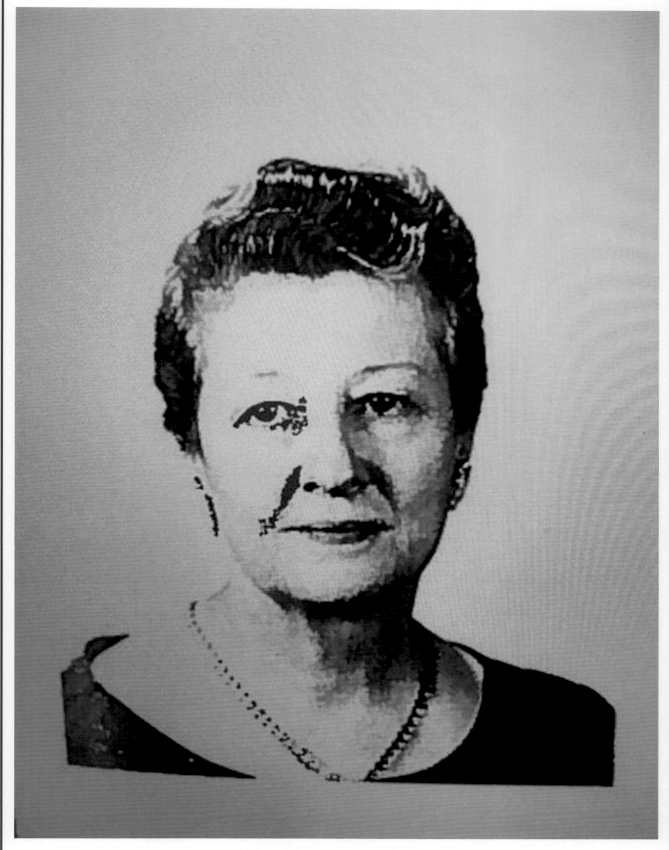

ETHEL B. SAGER

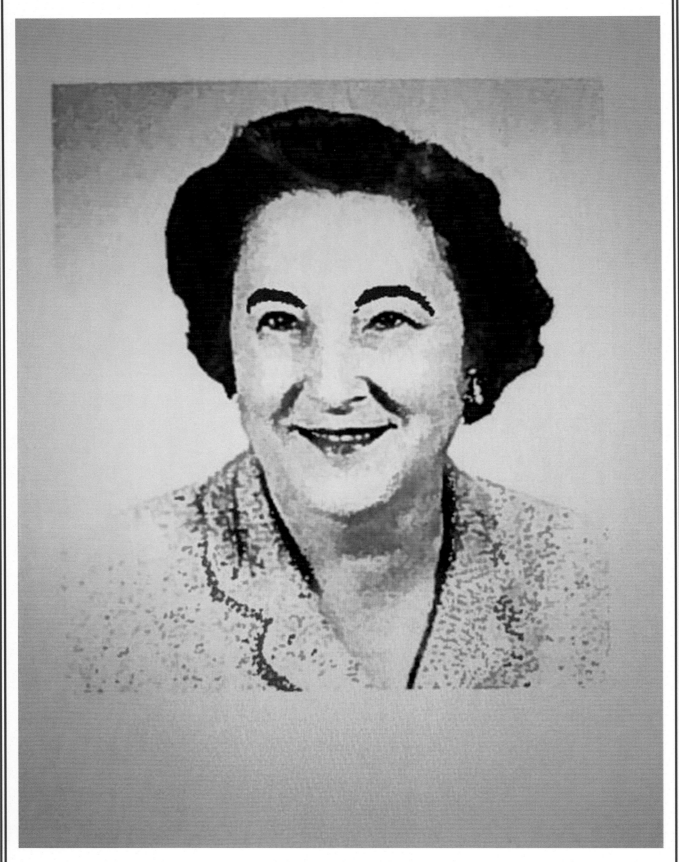

HELEN BRAUN

While in high school I read a novel about a heroic psychiatrist who became obsessed with a young, beautiful schizophrenic woman. He dedicated himself to delving like a detective into her earlier life and discovering the "trauma" that caused her break from reality. Of course, new anti-psychotic drugs had just appeared as adjuncts to counseling schizophrenics, but they only played a supportive role. In any case, I decided right then that I wanted to replay this novel in person, but it turned out to be as fictional in real life as it was in the book. In order to be a psychiatrist, it was necessary to go to medical school to become an MD. Of course, I romanticized the whole thing, as I was prone to do.

I had quite an experience at Cornell, but not necessarily the one I expected. As a result, I have urged my 4 children, with limited success, to attend a good, but not necessarily large and prestigious, (and obscenely expensive,) undergraduate college. My three daughters followed my advice, at least to the extent of avoiding large schools, but my son went to NYU where he majored in music and advanced mathematics and enjoyed the big city life until he didn't.

Before matriculating at Cornell, I had already decided that I wanted to go to medical school to become a psychiatrist. Although I had no experience with psychiatrists or psychotherapy, (although I certainly needed it,) I was heavily influenced by emotional problems of my own related to a dysfunctional, if well -meaning family, and the need to be loved (and useful).

Once at Cornell, I signed up for courses to major in English and minor in Art History while taking the minimum number of courses required for medical school, so minimum that I could only apply to a fraction of medical schools. I did not know that at the time nor was I advised otherwise. I do not think this would have happened at a smaller more personalized school.

I was a fair English major, and my writing ability, (you be the judge,) vastly improved out of necessity, a better and more inspired art history minor, but barely got by in my science courses for which I had little enthusiasm. One exception was my course in comparative anatomy taught by an expert on sharks, Dr. Perry Webster Gilbert, whom I found fascinating and inspirational. I also loved physics and still do. I believe physics, strange as it might seem, to be the most spiritual of all the sciences. I say that because even Einstein admitted that even physics in its most profound elegance cannot explain how and from where it all started. I remember our flamboyant professor, in front of several hundred students, demonstrating the pendular movement of a heavy iron ball hanging from the ceiling, walking the ball as far as possible to one side and handing it to an assistant, then counting paces back to the mirror image spot in the pathway of the ball, closing his eyes, and commanding that the ball be released. Of course, the ball touched his head, very gently, and the point was made.

Chemistry, both inorganic and organic, was not my cup of bromine. I dropped organic chemistry when I discovered that it required a two-hour lab session every Saturday morning at 8 a.m. which interfered with my social agenda. Instead, I took the course at Columbia U. over the summer while I also framed a house with my college roommate for his architect brother in Rye, NY. This started me thinking about architecture, a clue that maybe medicine was not for me, but my father was adamant that I must be a doctor, and I capitulated. It might be of some interest that one of the most memorable of all my childhood experiences was seeing an exhibit of Van Gogh's works at the Toledo Art

Museum. My mother painted, but was discouraged by my father who, a mechanical engineer, saw little value in such things. Later, when I had the audacity to consider a career in architecture instead of medicine, my father predictably and successfully intervened. Ironically, my first cousin and childhood chum, Sam Davis, who lived across the street, eventually became the Dean of Architecture at U.C. Berkeley. He has left a legacy in the Bay Area of developing good housing for have-nots such as the homeless, HIV-afflicted, and international students without the means to afford decent housing.

While at Cornell, I joined a fraternity, Phi Sigma Kappa, because many of my fellow members of the Cornell rowing team joined the same fraternity. This turned out to be a very socially conservative fraternity which originated in the south. I believe I was its first Jew and later discovered that there had never been a black member. At my initiation, chapter officers wore hoods that were similar to those associated with the Ku Klux Klan. I ultimately became the Chapter President which gave me a platform for reform. We managed to recruit the chapter's first African American member despite some very disturbing bigotry on full display during the recruitment process. Later, as a member of the Cornell Interfraternity Council, I participated in the trial of a fraternity which had exercised verbal abuse upon a black student at one of its parties. I became acquainted with a group of disenchanted black students who later took over the Student Union building during the racial unrest that occurred in 1968. I also became acquainted with Sandy Berger who was President of the IFC and later served as Bill Clinton's Chief-of-Staff; he was a brilliant and inspirational young man, who, like me, was unsuccessful in assisting the Black Justice Movement on campus. Unfortunately, things have changed very little since then as the current racial protests indicate.

This brings up the issue of my college social life which is worth mentioning if only briefly because I am in good company when it comes to 18 year-old males who waste much of their undergraduate college experience seeking fun of which they were largely deprived during high school while trying too hard to please parents and get into the "best schools". Much of the social seeking was for "love", of which I felt deprived in my youth.

I found love, eventually, in the person of Irene Caldwell, a devout Catholic. Our relationship was equally and insensitively denounced both by the Catholic Church and by my Reform rabbi, but we found a renegade priest who married us, shortly after I was graduated, in a ceremony in which half the church was occupied by Jews and the other, Catholics. My Polish mother-in-law- of blessed memory, also Irene, broke her promise and managed to sneak in a singer of faith to perform an operatic version of Ave Maria as we walked the isle. Later that day, while having a reception in Irene's back yard in New Hyde Park, Long Island under a tent, a sudden cloudburst ominously occurred, and we were all drenched. There endeth our ill-fated wedding, June 25, 1967—divorced 1984.

Once safely married, we were off to Lake Placid, New York where we both lost our virginity, with each other, and had a wonderful first summer of marriage. I ran my father's fudge shop, and Irene kept house. I learned to fly fish, and we saw plays. We were visited by my aging maternal grandfather, Alex Zinn, very charming and shamelessly cheap, a former boxer in the era of Jewish boxers, whose career was ended when he lost an eye, something I am certain was predicted by his Jewish mother since many Jewish mothers have been known to say, "Don't go outside or play sports; you could put an eye out!". We also spent time with my great aunt Jenny Koenigsberg whose husband, Joseph Koenigsberg was related to Woody Allen " Koenigsberg". Jenny, after whom my first child was named, was a beautiful and elegant lady of Jewish/Austrian descent who was one of many women in her family who were well educated for their time and many of whom became teachers, the profession most revered by Jews. Two of my children, Jennifer and Rebecca, work in childhood education. Jennifer, a Harvard graduate, works in educational reform, while Rebecca helped start an innovative school in Stowe, Vermont in which much of the learning occurs outdoors where lessons are learned from nature.

Unfortunately, that otherwise idyllic summer was scarred by the untimely death of my favorite uncle, Allen Rosenberg, in an auto accident that still carries great mystery and pain. His was the first personal death I ever experienced, but only the beginning. He was sober, good weather, daylight, under financial pressure. His wife, my aunt Dorothy, was eventually re-married to a wealthy man who never ingratiated himself to my family. Uncle Allen, along with my father and Uncle Maury who was married to my father's sister Isabel, used to be outrageous pranksters at family events, sometimes quite off-color. Dorothy's new spouse never joined the club. This death of a loved one was very traumatic for me since Allen was often more of a father to me than my own; he used to hold me by the feet and shake money out of me which was mine to keep of course. We rolled side-by-side down the hills of Cincinnati where he lived until I was ready to vomit, but laughing as I had never laughed at home.

Once this memorable summer ended, Irene and I were off to Philadelphia where I had managed to squeak into medical school at Hahnemann Medical College, now Drexel University Medical College. I was married, motivated, and did very well in medical school where

I was graduated in the top 10% of my class and a member of AOA Medical Society, the medical equivalent of Phi Beta Kappa.

In my third year, which is the first year of clinical rotations, I did my psychiatry rotation at the famous Philadelphia General Hospital which had a large unit for the institutionalized insane. There I did not see anything that vaguely resembled the book that had inspired my interest in psychiatry. These patients were too delusional, although often very interesting in their delusions, to carry on any useful counselling. Their treatment, essentially palliative, was to give them powerful anti-psychotic medications. Furthermore, my first two years of work in medical school had engendered a real interest in the science of medicine. I was very inspired by my pediatric rotation despite losing my first patient, a beautiful teenaged woman with Marfan's syndrome who died suddenly when her aorta burst. I visited with her one day, then discovered the next that she had died. Like the first of just about everything, this experience has stuck, but, inexplicably, only strengthened my interest in pediatrics.

During my fourth year, having already determined to continue my post-doctoral training in pediatrics, I had an elective in pediatric-hematology-oncology at St. Christopher's Hospital for Children which was part of Temple University's medical school. I was mentored by Dr. J. Lawrence "Lawry" Naiman, a great teacher among many others who were on staff there at that halcyon time. The whole experience at St. Chris was transformative as many of the faculty were superstars in their various areas of interest. The most important experience, however, as it related to my future plans, was a weekly teaching session with Dr. Naiman which he held each Friday morning. He set up a number of microscopes showing blood slides from patients about whom these slides, if properly examined, were informative and often diagnostic.

We were given a bit of history and asked to systematically examine the slides and answer questions which often led to the diagnosis of complex diseases simply by looking at a slide and learning as much from it as possible. We were assisted on site by Lawry's fellow, Dr. Howard Schmuckler, an unfortunate name which, if you know Yiddish, likens you to the male sex organ in a most unflattering way. I am a visual learner, (and later discovered that I am a visual artist,) so this experience of actually visualizing the pathology was seminal and also prophetic, and I quickly resolved to pursue the study of pediatric hematology-oncology which required first that I become a pediatrician.

Since I loved children, pediatrics seemed ideal until I later realized that I disliked the daily tasks of a general pediatrician profoundly, especially the issue of infant feeding, in comparison to the opportunity to diagnose and treat the more challenging and life-threatening illnesses of childhood which are rare in a general pediatric practice. I was aware that the choice of pediatric medicine meant less income and prestige neither of which I thought much about even though I had become a father, (Jennifer Lynn, DOB 2/13/70,) in my third year of medical school.

So there you have the somewhat convoluted, but not unique story of how I got into medicine to begin with and how my plans changed completely during the process. One lesson to be taken from all this is that I had (have) a need to be "useful" as explained in the prelude to this book. Here the word useful understates a drive to stand out from the crowd and to take on difficult challenges and, in the process, to earn admiration if not love. I also now realize that I was (am) more an artist than a scientist at heart, but was ultimately able to practice medicine as if it were a blank canvas full of colors, lines, and textures, made up by real people with real problems.

It would be another 35 years before I started painting in earnest at the advice of a therapeutic Watsu instructor who told me that I needed to get in touch with my right brain more and suggested painting with my non-dominant left hand (which I don't do or need to do). She so advised me after a one hour water therapy session during which I was blindfolded and moved through the warm water with floaters on my feet so that the brilliant therapist could hold my head and upper body in order to go through a routine of gentle stretches and positions, all noise drowned out by the water. From this she was able to draw the correct conclusion about my need to access my right brain with its daring and creativity to compliment my left brained, (mostly I hope,) evidence-based medical practice. I have become a respectable painter with the support and savvy of my more talented wife Aura. I use much color and movement in my predominantly abstract works and plan to pursue art more once retired, hopefully soon, if ever. I believe I approached my patients with art in mind most of the time as I hope you will see in the following pages.

I applied to a few places to continue my training and landed, fortuitously I believe, in Denver, Colorado at Children's Hospital where we will spend most of the next chapter.

CHAPTER 3

I Recount My Internship and Residency in Pediatrics and My Early Transition to a Fellowship in Pediatric Blood and Cancer

I chose Denver over locations in California for my pediatric training because there was something very appealing to me about the Children's Hospital and the Rocky Mountains. I had never lived anywhere except the east coast and Ohio and was looking for something new and exciting as well as the excellent education.

At that time, the pediatric training program in Denver consisted of three hospitals, Children's, Colorado General (University) Hospital, and Denver General Hospital. The University component at Colorado General Hospital was highly regarded nationally. Children's had a full-time staff of professors, but was less academic and accommodated the many local pediatricians who wanted to follow their own hospitalized patients, a practice that no longer exists, at least in cities. Colorado General was the elite hub stuffed with many stalwarts in various disciplines led by the estimable Dr. C. Henry Kemp, a true advocate for battered children along with Fred Battaglia and Lula Lubchenko, two brilliant neonatologists. Denver General was an inner-city hospital with limited resources, but a wealth of challenging patients from which to learn. I was based at Children's where I found the more approachable faculty and less self-impressed trainees.

This tripartite system was hierarchical and led to some difficulties. For example, Dr. Battaglia came to Children's weekly to conduct rounds in its newborn intensive care unit for which he had little respect. Neonatology was a part of pediatrics that I dreaded. I literally never slept a wink on my schedule of 36 hours on and 12 off, all in the name of continuity of care for the sick newborns, but physically and emotionally barbaric. Furthermore, he would arrive about 7 a.m. after we had been up all night doing meaningless, but necessary tasks that could have been done and are now done better by the nursing staff. He grilled us on trivia such as the rate of head growth in a baby that could not be taken out of its incubator to be measured because of respiratory distress. If we didn't know the answers, we were maligned as if we were perpetrators of the infant's imminent demise.

Dr. Battaglia, "affectionately" known at the Bat Man, was much feared, but also respected for his considerable contributions to a burgeoning field. However, there is much in neonatology that struck me as ethically ambiguous. It is a field where the ability to keep very premature babies alive, despite often bearing severe congenital birth defects or other conditions with limited prospects for meaningful survival, took precedence over the end result for child and family. Once the technology was there, it was very difficult not to use it and to know where to draw the line. There was much to be learned, however, especially about blood which was beneficial to me in future pursuits.

Neonatology was my first and most traumatic clinical rotation. I returned home one night after working without sleep for 36 hours where my wife had prepared a lobster dinner for our anniversary. I promptly fell asleep at the table with my face planted in the unfortunate crustacean. Mercifully, the practice of keeping residents sleep-deprived and then grilling them on trivia in the pre-dawn gloom, a form of hazing I believe, has been discontinued and a premium placed on thinking and learning. I didn't harbor any animosity for Dr. Battaglia, only his medieval philosophy of teaching by fear and bullying which might suit the military, but not aspiring pediatricians, (perhaps the most docile of all medical stereotypes). I learned a great deal, but this experience served to accelerate my zeal to get to what I really wanted to do in pediatrics, namely hematology/oncology.

We did have some fun notwithstanding my lack of enthusiasm for general pediatrics. Dr. Henry Sondheimer, who eventually became a pediatric cardiologist, was my supervisory resident, and we were covering the infectious disease unit. It was Halloween, and we decided to play a prank on our attending infectious disease physician, Dr. McIntosh, a generally jovial man, but one who was formal and stiff when teaching. This made him an ideal target for our plan.

We obtained a large pumpkin and carved it to look like it was taking its last breath. We put the pumpkin in a mist tent in a private room and fogged up the tent so that nothing could be seen inside it. We had a chart prepared in medical records and sent tap water for a urinalysis to make it look official. On rounds, we told Dr. McIntosh that this patient looked a little yellow and had a diagnosis of epiglottitis, an extremely dangerous infection of the throat which can obstruct breathing and cause death. Such patients should never be out of sight and often require a breathing tube. Upon hearing this story, delivered with perfectly straight faces, Dr. McIntosh got a look of horror on his face, ran into the room, literally ripped the tent off the bed, and discovered the pumpkin with an intravenous line running into it. He quickly realized that he had been "played", but was so upset that he could not continue rounds.

We took him to the doctors' lounge where he eventually regained his composure after drinking some coffee.

At that time, but no longer, it was permissible to begin a sub-specialty fellowship in the third year of pediatrics instead of continuing with general pediatrics. I jumped at the opportunity and began my fellowship in the summer of 1973. My first mentor was Dr. Charles August, (see photo in Chapter 5) a tweedy Harvard graduate who was trained in pediatric hematology at the Boston Children's Hospital under Louis Diamond and David Nathan, two towering figures in the field who also trained my mentor at UCLA, Dr. Stephen Feig, where I would complete my fellowship after a two- year hiatus in the Army Medical Corps. Since Charles had planned a vacation just as I was starting, he sent me to Aspen, Colorado where there was an excellent seminar in immunology at the Given Institute.

I spent my days learning from many of the world's smartest clinical immunologists and scientists, and my evenings tying flies and fly fishing. It was one of the best of all training experiences and gave me a break from my domestic responsibilities as well. This experience initiated an interest in immunobiology that has served me well throughout my career. Charles, therefore, is *mensch* number 3.

Charles and I managed to write my first published paper in which we reported the treatment of hemolytic-uremic syndrome with drugs that inhibited the function of blood platelets which we postulated were being deposited in and damaging the kidneys and other sites. We believed that "poisoning" the platelets with these drugs might slow or stop the process. We were partially correct as it turned out, and we probably contributed to a better understanding of this unusual disease. Sadly, Charles,"Chas", passed away 3 years ago after a distinguished career.

After my hematology rotation, it was time to work with cancer patients under the leadership of Dr. Charlene Holton, now Holt. She was trained at St. Jude's Hospital for Children in Tennessee which is famously supported by philanthropy initiated by comedian Danny Thomas from my home town of Toledo, Ohio and continued by his daughter Marlo Thomas, also a television celebrity. At that time, St. Jude's was one of a select group of centers that focused on childhood cancer. Charlene was well trained and well connected. She inspired me with her single-mindedness and, yes, Courage. She is *mensch* number 4.

These were the daunting early days of the field of childhood cancer. We had few tools either to successfully treat the disease or reduce the suffering of the children. Many very capable people entered the field and found that they couldn't bear it. Others, like me, stayed because we correctly believed that things would get better, because they couldn't get worse. We were right.

What we did have and needed were each other's backs. Charlene astutely arranged weekly meetings with a psychologist, Dr. Chet Peremba, in which we were given an opportunity to ventilate and encourage our tight little group to stay the course. During the time that I was in the group, a movie was made featuring an experience that Charlene had with a teenaged girl with bone cancer who refused amputation, the only treatment available at the time, and died. The movie included a beautiful actress playing the part of Charlene, who was herself a beautiful young woman, and featured the music of John Denver who was at the peak of his career and a fellow Coloradan. We all went to see him at Red Rocks Amphitheater, a spectacular outdoor venue in Denver, and had a powerful bonding experience. This was the closest I have ever been to a group of fellow caregivers, and was, despite the tragedies that we dealt with daily, truly exhilarating. My interest moved from hematology to oncology during these few months and never changed.

During this rotation, Dr. John Hutter, one of the junior faculty members, and I encountered a patient with neuroblastoma, one of the common solid tumors of childhood, whose father had the same disease and survived, (also the outcome of our patient). We published our observation and found other cases in the literature. A few years later, Dr. Alfred "Two Hit" Knudson, husband of a well- known pediatric oncologist, Dr. Anna Meadows, published a paper describing the exceptional cases of hereditary neuroblastoma and other hereditary tumors as a "two hit" phenomenon whereby a child inherits a cancer gene from a parent, but a second mutation (genetic event) of variable frequency is needed to cause the cancer. Retinoblastoma, a childhood tumor of the eye, is the classic example of this phenomenon in which a child who inherits the retinoblastoma gene will develop retinoblastoma with a frequency of 90%. Non-hereditary cancers require at least two infrequent mutations and are, therefore, much less likely to occur than their hereditary counterparts. Of course, now we understand that numerous cancers, mostly of adults, have an underlying genetic risk factor, but in these early days, hereditary cancer was new information.

Lorrie Odom, another pediatric oncologist who would be my department chairman when I finally returned to Denver in 1988, was just finishing her training at St. Jude's at the time. When she returned, she treated and cured a patient of leukemia at age 14 that I am now following in her 50s for complications of part of her treatment, brain radiation, which was given to prevent relapse of leukemia in the brain. Under my care, I have treated her for both secondary benign brain tumors as well as visual loss related to previous brain radiation which we reversed with hyperbaric oxygen therapy (HBOT). This treatment will be discussed in detail in a later chapter.

Other important team members at that time were Gail Levine, pediatric pathologist, Jack Chang, pediatric surgeon, and Mary Jo Cleveland, pediatric oncology nurse. These fine people would all become part of my life again years later and all had an early impact. Jack Chang is honored in detail in the next chapter as Mensch number 5 of eighteen described in this text. Gail came back into my life when I saw her present her poetry and signed up with her to help me with mine which she did (with limited success). Mary Jo was Director of pediatric oncology nursing at Children's Hospital when I returned to Denver in 1988.

Shortly after these events, I departed to serve in the Army Medical Corps during the latter part of the Viet Nam War, but before I end this chapter, I should mention an anecdote of some interest. While I was doing my oncology rotation, two of the more senior fellows, whose names shall not be mentioned for obvious reasons, apparently fell in love although already married. One night when they were on call together, they mysteriously disappeared for a few hours and couldn't be reached. Soon thereafter, one of the surgical fellows also disappeared while on call. During his disappearance, no one could reach the breathy-voiced solo night operator at Children's Hospital. Fortunately, no harm was done to the patients during these escapades. I guess the take home message is that no matter how difficult things get in medicine, there is always the need and possibility of love, if that's what we choose to call it. I guess, in most cases, that is a good thing.

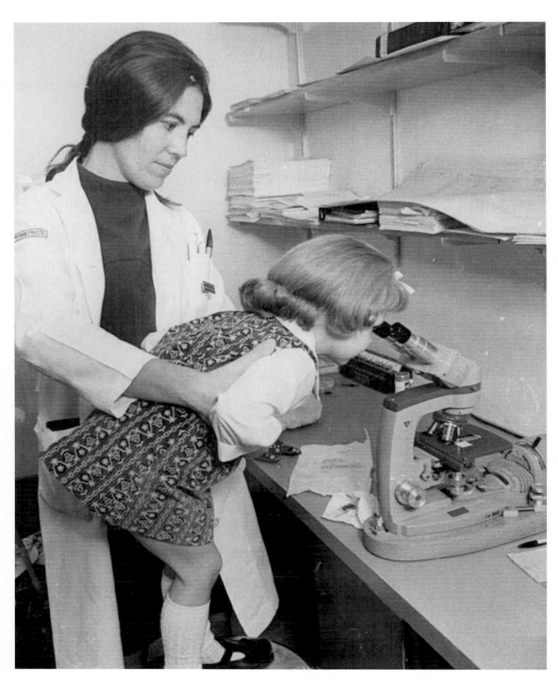

DR. CHARLENE HOLTON
Purchased from Getty Imaging

CHAPTER 4

The Conquest Of Childhood Cancer

A Milestone in the History of Medicine

When I started my fellowship in pediatric hematology-oncology in 1973, the same year that I became an avid birder, childhood leukemia and most other childhood malignancies were fatal diseases with very short survival. Our treatment armamentarium was limited to surgery, primitive radiation therapy, and a few chemotherapeutic agents. These agents included vincristine, one of three drugs derived from the vinca plant which prevents tumor cell division, actinomycin D, which is produced by bacteria in culture and inhibits tumor cell protein function, corticosteroids which poison malignant cells of the immune system, methotrexate which blocks activation of the vitamin folic acid upon which some tumor cells are dependent, and mercaptopurine which poisons tumor cell DNA.

We did not have good anti-nausea drugs, no central venous access, no conscious sedation for procedures, no adequate or safe source of blood platelets, no means of preventing or treating chicken pox which was often fatal, no prevention or adequate treatment for pneumocystis, a life-threatening lung infection, no drugs to hasten recovery of blood cells from chemotherapy, and inadequate means of controlling pain. The task of caring for these children and consoling parents was formidable, and many very smart and well-intentioned people could not bear it. I did, but I'm not sure how.

In order to keep going in this context, it was necessary to have a team of caregivers who provided mutual support. As opposed to other cultures, such as Russia, where a cancer diagnosis was often misrepresented to patients and parents, we tried to be truthful and compassionate at the same time and expressed hope that answers were forthcoming. Other than the emotional burden, there was very little pressure. We had little to lose, and we had not caused the disease. At least we were willing to try, and that gave us a certain *esprit de corps* from which we derived motivation. What we could provide was compassion and empathy which we did, often with substantial emotional cost. Essentially, things couldn't be worse, so they must get better, or so we believed, but this belief was based more on faith than fact. We could not accept that things would not improve; we were right.

Let me begin with Wilms tumor, a childhood kidney cancer which is the most common solid tumor of childhood. Former US Attorney General and pediatric surgeon C. Everett Koop, had a particular interest in this disease. This tumor was seldom found before it was large and surgically incurable and/or had already spread to regional lymph nodes and/or beyond and was thus, at the time, incurable. With surgery or surgery plus local radiation, cures were about 10%, and all other patients died of their disease. In the 1960s, Drs. Audrey Evans and Giulio D'Angio from Children's Hospital of Philadelphia, along with Dr. Koop and a handful of other visionary pediatric oncologists, formed a group which they called the National Wilms Tumor Study, NWTS, affectionately referred to by people in the field as NitWits. To the best of my knowledge, this was the first cancer consortium and the forerunner of many others. By pooling resources, including patients and professionals, this group was able to conduct meaningful clinical trials, one of which permanently changed the paradigm for cancer treatment from PALLIATION, which was focused on symptom control and extension of survival with minimal risk, to INTENT TO CURE which employed a strategy for eradication of the cancer which often involved substantial risk.

Before NWTS, chemotherapy was utilized timidly as single agent therapy in which a drug was chosen and given until, predictably, it stopped working or was excessively toxic at which point another drug, if any were available, would be added. The idea was to limit side effects and risk and save something for later. This approach and philosophy are still in common use, particularly in adults, but, as we would discover, never lead to cure.

Combining toxic drugs at a time of limited ability to manage toxicity was daunting, but the logical next step if cure was the goal, and it was. Thus, the NWTS, with full support of Drs. D'Angio, Evans, and other stalwarts, designed a study for Wilms tumor in which vincristine and actinomycin D were given singly or in combination in a prospective randomized trial. It took a few years to realize what had happened-- children who were "doomed" were surviving and ultimately found to be cured. The curability of Wilms rose to nearly 90%, and deaths primarily occurred in subsets with features which predicted lower survival. I can't emphasize enough how crucial this observation was to the future of cancer treatment. A number of other virulent malignancies including childhood leukemia and Hodgkin's disease in both children and adults as well as some non-Hodgkin's lymphomas soon became curable and led to a flurry of activity to find the safest and most effective drug COMBINATIONS.

This dramatic development in cancer treatment was predicted by the tuberculosis experience in which only combinations of antibiotics and never single drugs led to cure and nearly eradicated the disease. Cancer has turned out to be a much more formidable challenge, and cure remains elusive for many, especially the most common malignancies of adults, despite the early successes with combination chemotherapy in children.

Let me return to and dwell on childhood leukemia, acute lymphoblastic leukemia (ALL). At the time of my own childhood and early days of medical education, just hearing the word, leukemia, brought about a visceral response of fear and revulsion. Two of my classmates in elementary school died of ALL. My brief stint as a practicing pediatrician taught me that parents feared this disease as much or more than anything else that could happen to their children once the polio vaccine became available. Although relatively rare, it was the most common malignancy of childhood and universally fatal. Death was not only certain, but came quickly and with great suffering.

Sydney Farber, one of the early physicians to tackle this disease, and after whom the Dana-Farber Cancer Institute at Harvard is named, gave patients supplemental vitamins in a desperate effort to keep them from literally wasting away as the disease chewed up calories and tissues. He and others noted that the use of nutritional supplementation caused the progress of the disease to accelerate (this experience now forms the best argument for discouraging patients from using nutrition as a treatment for cancer in the absence of strong scientific evidence). Farber honed in on the B vitamin folic acid which was known to be crucial for normal production of blood cells by the bone marrow and the deficiency of which could produce severe underproduction of all blood cells including white blood cells.

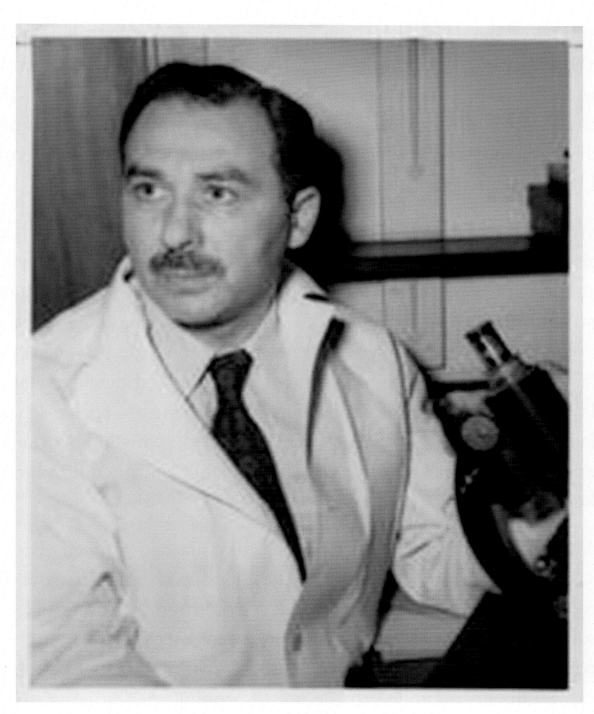

SYDNEY FARBER MD
Obtained with permission to publish from Boston Children's Hospital

Investigations confirmed that childhood leukemic cells, which were immature lymphocytes, had a requirement for folic acid in order to proliferate and survive. This knowledge led to the development of a drug, aminopterin, a predecessor of methotrexate, both of which are inhibitors of the enzyme tetrahydrofolate reductase which is required for the activation of dietary folic acid. Activated folic acid is a necessary cofactor for DNA biosynthesis. Methotrexate and other drugs that interfere with DNA replication are known as anti-metabolites, a family of chemotherapy drugs which are especially effective against leukemias and lymphomas, cancers of blood cell origin.

Methotrexate was effective enough in childhood leukemia to achieve remission in some patients, a state in which the blood count returns to normal and the bone marrow is grossly rid of leukemic cells. Unfortunately, these remissions were temporary as we would have predicted based on the Wilms tumor story if we had known it at the time. As mentioned earlier, mercaptopurine, another anti-metabolite, had been developed, and we knew that leukemia would respond transiently to corticosteroids and vincristine. Once these drugs were combined, remission became the rule rather than the exception, and the challenge morphed into how to make the remission permanent.

Physicians caring for children with leukemia had noticed that the first site of relapse was not always the blood and bone marrow, but often the central nervous system and, less commonly, the testicles. A reasonable postulate was that these sites were somehow "sanctuaries" where leukemic cells could escape the therapeutic effects of systemic therapy. This postulate led to the use of prophylactic radiation to the whole brain. This innovation, which took courage given the suspected (and underestimated) vulnerability of the developing brain to radiation, along with the addition of L-asparaginase to the armamentarium, a drug which lowered the levels of an amino acid required by leukemic cells, led to something that was literally unimaginable just a few years earlier, the CURE of childhood leukemia.

Ultimately, we found safer ways than radiation to prevent central nervous system relapse for most patients with ALL. Along with the cure of tuberculosis, discovery of microbes as the cause of human infectious disease, the discovery of effective antibiotics, especially penicillin, and vaccines, the cure of childhood leukemia and other childhood cancers through the use of combination chemotherapy stands out as one of the great achievements in the history of medicine, and the use of combination chemotherapy instead of serial single agents became and remains the prototype for curing cancer. Dr. Vincent DaVita, best known for curing Hodgkin's Disease with combination chemotherapy, authored an authoritative textbook of medical oncology, entitled CANCER: Principles and Practice of Oncology, in which he states that cancer cannot be cured with single agent chemotherapy, but only when effective combinations are developed. This book in in its eleventh edition, and this statement has never changed.

Once it was recognized that ALL was curable, efforts escalated, very understandably, to make the treatment safer and less intrusive to the normal life of a child. Dr. D'Angio famously and prophetically proclaimed, "cure is not enough, we must fix the damage". One study sought, for patients with ALL classified as low risk for relapse, to give less aggressive and potentially safer treatment. Patients were randomly assigned to standard treatment vs something less. One of my first patients after I became Section Head of Pediatric Hem-Onc. at Albany Medical College was on this study and was randomized to the less aggressive arm. She relapsed early, responded poorly to second line treatment, and died.

I was devastated and was present for her death along with her despondent family. We all thought, but didn't state the obvious question:

would it have been otherwise if she had gotten the standard treatment? Of course, we will never know the answer to this haunting question. What I can say is that the study was closed prematurely because of an excess of failures in the less aggressive arm. Some children, possibly including my patient, gave their lives to gain this valuable knowledge. This experience contributed to my future behavior as a risk-taker who preferred to give more rather than less in the context of life-threatening illnesses. It also led, perhaps by serendipity, to a great interest in finding ways to prevent or correct the damage done by otherwise successful therapy without compromising the therapy itself.

About the same time that I had the traumatic experience detailed above, another major event was brewing in the childhood cancer saga. One of the most public, but rare childhood and young adult cancers, (about 800 cases per year in US), was a bone tumor called osteosarcoma (OS). It was the disease that took the life of a famous University of Texas football player named Freddie Steinmark and very similar to the bone cancer that one of the Kennedy children had and survived. This cancer was most common in teenagers and young adults. It was the subject of a movie made for television in the early 70s during my first year of hematology-oncology training that I mentioned in an earlier chapter.

Later, this disease began to yield to aggressive and innovative use of chemotherapy which was necessary to prevent the nearly universal and fatal spread of the tumor, predominantly to the lungs. Dr. Gerald Rosen, at Memorial Sloan-Kettering Cancer Center in New York, pioneered the use of very high dose methotrexate to treat OS. He taught me how to do this safely as I was close by in Albany and a collaborator. The trick of safely giving what otherwise would have been lethal doses of methotrexate was to "rescue" the patient with an antidote which was simply the active form of the vitamin folic acid which methotrexate blocked. This was greatly facilitated by the ability to get blood methotrexate levels done quickly in the laboratory to guide the "rescue". Patients received doses of methotrexate that were 600-1000 times the dose that we gave children weekly for leukemia, with few or no significant adverse side effects. Without an antidote, this was a lethal dose. Gerald even figured out how to give this therapy as an outpatient to avoid prolonged stays in the hospital while the methotrexate levels gradually declined to a safe level in an otherwise asymptomatic patient.

To make a long story short, this therapy clearly improved survival for patients with osteosarcoma and reduced or delayed spread to the lungs and other sites. Other chemotherapy using the drugs cisplatin and doxorubicin showed great promise, and consideration was given to trying to avoid amputation. At the same time, the Mayo Clinic published institutional data which seemed to indicate that chemotherapy added little or nothing to amputation and showed survival using early amputation alone which was better than others had observed. Heated debates took place which led, ultimately, to an ill-fated randomized clinical trial in one of the pediatric consortia comparing amputation alone vs amputation and chemotherapy. This study was stopped within less than one year because of excessive deaths from progressive disease in the surgery only arm.

I, as head of my program in Albany, had made the executive decision, based on personal experience, not to participate. I had learned my lesson the hard way, and it paid off. Another lesson from this story is not to rely on single institution experiences, no matter how prestigious the institution. Once again, lives were lost for science, but not in vain. Those few who did not survive have saved the lives of many subsequent patients. If any readers of this book were friends or family of any of those who died tragically to prove this point, I want to make sure that they know that their loved ones have not been forgotten, and that they live on in the lives of those that have been saved by their sacrifice.

The osteosarcoma story does not end here. About 10 years later, I found myself back in Denver at the old Children's Hospital where I had the good fortune to work with Dr. John Cullen and his wife Patsy McGuire Cullen PhD CPNP who is now Assistant Dean for Graduate Nursing Programs at Regis University in Denver. This couple had a particular interest in and worked together to improve the outcome for patients with pediatric bone tumors including osteosarcoma. John and Patsy, along with Dr. Tom Smith, joined me and others in our exodus from Children's to Presbyterian St. Luke's Medical Center in about 1992. There we had the opportunity to work with the Center for Limb Preservation headed by a visionary orthopedic surgeon, Dr. Ross Wilkins, who along with Dr. Kyle Fink, a medical oncologist, were using an innovative treatment for osteosarcoma in which intra-arterial cisplatin was infused directly into the primary bone tumor along with systemic intravenous doxorubicin.

This approach was hatched in Boston by Dr. Norman Jaffe and continued at MD Anderson Cancer Center in Houston by Dr. Robert Benjamin. Dr. Cullen successfully reduced the frequency and severity of mucous membrane breakdown by reducing the infusion time of the doxorubicin from 72 to 48 hours. This is an example of how simple, but carefully considered modifications can make major differences in outcome. In this case, the change resulted in a shorter hospital stay and fewer cases of infection, both attributable to reduced injury to mucous membranes from mouth to anus.

Serial arteriograms demonstrated progressive loss of the dramatically increased blood supply to these tumors. Once there was essentially no blood supply remaining, the tumors were invariably reduced in size enough to allow Dr. Wilkins to perform limb salvage surgery in which the mass, now essentially dead (necrotic), was removed and replaced with a graft of either cadaver or synthetic bone. The synthetic prostheses were able to expand as the patient grew so that they could be used before full height had been attained.

Two things of great importance were achieved by this approach. First, but still controversial, overall survival was better than survival achieved by primary amputation followed by systemic, but not intra-tumoral chemotherapy. The reason for this is unclear, but probably related to humoral factors released from the primary site that inhibited the growth of pulmonary metastases. Second, most patients were able to avoid amputation despite the challenges of adapting to major orthopedic intervention.

This experience was done at a single institution with a unique combination of innovative orthopedic surgery, oncology, and advanced oncology nursing, which would be difficult to replicate elsewhere. The approach requires extraordinary effort, expertise, and time. It is my sense as I write that this clearly superior approach has never become the standard approach that it should be, but perhaps understandably. My only role, other than to see the results first-hand, was to encourage my colleagues to persist in what was difficult and controversial. They did the same for me in my approach to childhood brain tumors which I will report in detail elsewhere in this book. John Cullen and I were kindred spirits in our commitment to the goal of cure for children with cancer and our willingness to take necessary risks in that pursuit.

This chapter, then, describes in detail, the monumental events which led to the cure of several cancers of childhood and provided a model for optimum treatment of cancer in general. Also described, and to be discussed in more detail later, is the phenomenon of a superior treatment being developed that, for a variety of reasons, never becomes standard and remains unavailable to many patients who could have benefitted from it, in some cases by surviving their otherwise fatal cancer.

In recalling these events from the perspective that I have forty years later, it strikes me that as my colleagues and I labored through these dramatic events, we did not fully comprehend their significance, namely that we had been participants in events that have saved thousands of lives and prevented immeasurable hardship to children and their families. Now, when I look back on those days, my eyes fill with tears of gratitude for the opportunity to have been "of use" in that miraculous time.

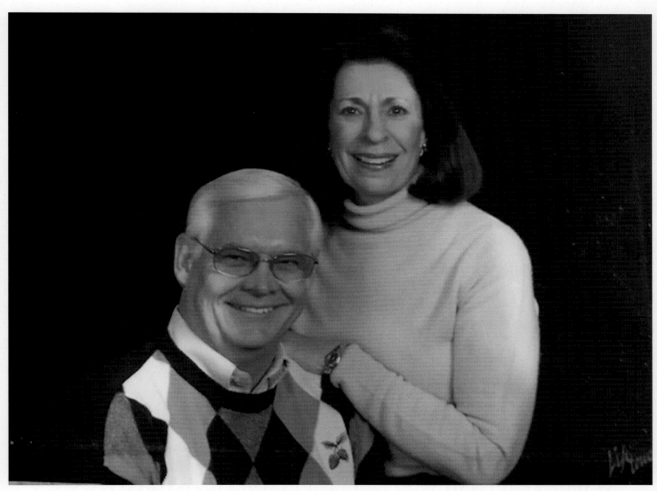

JOHN CULLEN MD AND PATSY CULLEN PhD CPNP

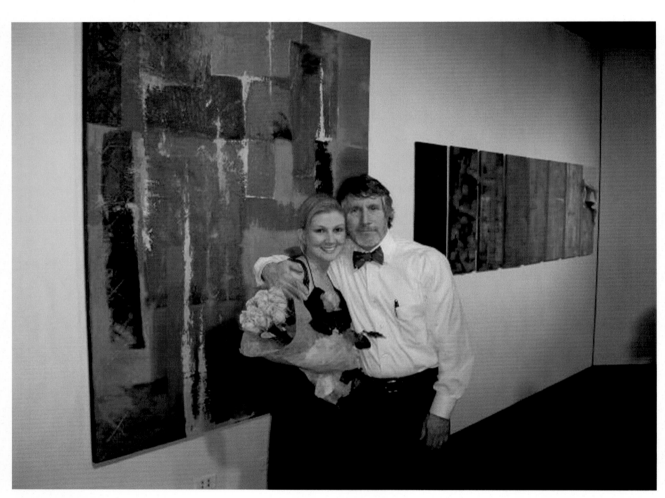

YOUR AUTHOR WITH THIRTY YEAR CHILDHOOD
CANCER SURVIVOR AND ARTIST KIMBERLEY BEESLEY

CHAPTER 5

Mensches 5, 6, and 7: Drs. Audrey Evans, Giulio D'Angio and a Cameo Appearance by Former Attorney General, Dr. C. Everett Koop

It might seem odd to include three individuals in one chapter, but none can be adequately described in the absence of the others. Together, working side-by-side at the Children's Hospital of Philadelphia, a part of the University of Pennsylvania, Drs. Evans, D'Angio, and Koop made huge contributions toward the cure of cancer as well as the prophetic recognition that successful treatment of cancer would create future problems for those fortunate enough to survive. While Dr. Evans was a pediatric oncologist, Dr. D'Angio was a pediatric radiation oncologist, both among the first (and best) in their fields. These two outstanding professionals also shared the experience of being rejected initially by American medical schools, Dr. D'Angio because he was an Italian immigrant, and Dr. Evans because she was a woman. They both quickly proved so talented that they broke through those barriers. Finally, theirs is a love story, well hidden from the public for many years although suspected. Their professional personas were so gracefully conducted that they were never, to the best of my knowledge, seen out of character by showing romantic affection for each other. Once retired, and in their 80s, they were married; their "secret" was finally out, much to the great joy of those who were lucky enough to know them.

Dr. D'Angio was born in 1922, and passed away in September, 2018. Dr. Evans, who was born in 1925 is still living. Dr. D'Angio is best known for his recognition of the damage caused by therapeutic radiation therapy and coining the statement "Cure is not enough. We must fix the damage". He also was a statesman who managed to facilitate the formation of the National Wilms Tumor Study which led to the cure of Wilms tumor and became a model for other cancer consortia. Dr. Evans developed a staging system for neuroblastoma and recognized, along with Dr. D'Angio and future Surgeon General C. Everett Koop, that some advanced neuroblastomas regress spontaneously and don't need treatment. She also is credited with establishing the first Ronald McDonald House, a home away from home for children with cancer and their families. I should also credit Dr. Koop with leading the fight against the tobacco industry while Surgeon General. These three giants collectively have probably contributed more to their respective fields than anyone else and with incomparable professionalism. I am privileged to have met and worked with them in my pediatric days.

Edward Arenson MD CWSP

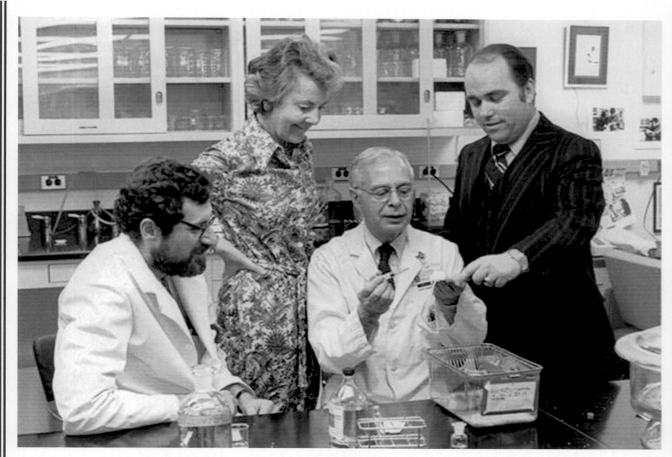

DRS. CHARLES AUGUST (SEE CHAPTER 3),
AUDREY EVANS, GIULIO D'ANGIO AND
UNIDENTIFIED PERSON IN SUIT
Photo obtained from Children's Hospital of
Philadelphia with permission to publish

CHAPTER 6

You're in the Army Now

I am writing on Monday, May 27, 2019; it is Memorial Day. I didn't always feel this way, but this is the most meaningful to me of all National Holidays with the possible exception of Mothers' Day. I believe it is worth telling the story of how I came to this point of view.

First, you must know where I started. I do not come from a military family, but my family has quite a history with the military. My father was of Lithuanian Jewish descent. His great-grandfather, Moses (Moshe) Sakilovsky, emigrated to the USA in the second half of the 19th Century to escape compulsory military service which had a very low expectation of survival for Jews. My great uncle, Edward Arenson, died in Europe in World War I. He is both my father's and my namesake. I am in possession of a copy of his last letter home. My cousin, Milford Myers, served in the Korean War and survived. He passed away in his 90s a couple of years ago and never seemed affected by his combat experience. My father was a Navy Lieutenant stationed in Philadelphia when I was born during World War II. He never saw combat because his skills as a Cornell-trained mechanical engineer were deemed more important than fighting. The night I was born at the Philadelphia Lying- In Hospital, a strictly maternity hospital, my father was intoxicated and admitted to a room near my mother's. I have never known him to be drunk since that night, but apparently his platoon was over-celebrating the departure of a most deplorable commanding officer. So that is the context of my inauspicious entry into the U.S. Army Medical Corps in the summer of 1974.

At the time, I had just completed the first year of a fellowship in Pediatric Hematology-Oncology at the Children's Hospital in Denver, Colorado. I had a wife and two very young children. In order to reduce my risk of being sent to Viet Nam, I enrolled in a program called the Berry Plan which would allow me to practice pediatrics during 2 years of military service, most likely stateside, but would interrupt my subspecialty training.

I tried to avoid this misfortune by applying for a position as a fellow in Pediatric Hem-Oncology at Walter Reed Army Medical Center in Bethesda, MD. I was accepted, but some higher-up made a decision that I was more needed at Fort Gordon, Georgia as a general pediatrician, a job I had already decided I would never do and which led to my early start as a subspecialist. It wasn't that I didn't like children. I had already accepted the reduced prestige and income that goes along with caring for children; the problem was that I wanted to deal with those children who were truly ill and in a medical field which represented one of the biggest of all challenges for children and adults, finding a cure for cancer. I simply had no interest in haggling with neurotic mothers over whether to breast feed or use formula and with cholic and all its pervasive emotional overlay. It had never been the kids that were the challenge, even when mortally ill; it was always their parents.

But it was not to be. I was sent to Augusta, Georgia, truly deep South, a place where the Ku Klux Klan was publicly active, the air stunk from pulp mills where wood was made into paper, and the weather was bitter cold in winter and stiflingly hot in summer. Many visualize the Augusta National

Golf Course with its gorgeous azaleas, blooming dogwoods, and brilliant green Bermuda grass fairways when they think of Augusta. I will tell you that the golf course, despite a long history of good old southern bigotry and misogyny, along with a wildlife preserve along the Savannah River, are the only beautiful things about Augusta other than its very hospitable and welcoming people. Perhaps it has changed, but I would be a hard sell.

To make the challenge a bit more complicated, I was a Yankee with all the expected biases against the South and Southern people. I grew up with an indignation about segregation, lost a Cornell classmate freedom rider in Mississippi, was on the liberal end of the political spectrum, and opposed the Viet Nam War and our obsession with the threat of communism, but I did have a sense of duty and patriotism that kept me out of the anti-war movement except at the ballot box.

I was also going through a medical education which can be all-consuming and leave little room for anything else. When I was an undergraduate at Cornell, my senior roommate would taunt me by putting up a poster of Nelson Rockefeller above my bed. Compared to the brand of Republican we see today, Nelson would be considered a gift from God. At that time, I was still grieving for JFK whose assassination was tolled by the college bells while I walked from the Cornell rowing tanks to my dorm. That is when I lost my childhood innocence and my belief that there might indeed be a better world for everyone. Perhaps I could contribute something during my lifetime that would make life better and/or longer for someone.

With all these misgivings about serving in the South, I made it clear to whomever assigned me there that I was no soldier, had low regard for the military, and would not be trained to be a soldier. I refused to attend training, got away with it, and showed up for duty totally unprepared. I managed to get my uniform and get signed in which takes a couple of days. However, when I showed up for my first day of work as a pediatrician, I was told by Sargent Jerry Bedicek, our NCO, that I was missing some badges and doodads from my uniform and therefore could not be seen until I got them or I would be in big trouble. He obviously knew what he was talking about, so I stayed in my office until he returned a few minutes later with everything I needed. I instinctively knew not to ask questions and didn't. Everything had turned out well.

Well, that is, until the Chief of Pediatrics, Major Frank Roberts, a cracker with limited medical skills, returned from leave and arrived late, as usual, for his monthly early morning department heads meeting. He put on his coat which had been hanging on a hook in his office and headed for his meeting. A few minutes later he returned to the clinic roaring for Sargent Bedicek, his ears as red as beefsteak tomatoes. He had arrived at his meeting out of uniform and was asked to leave. Of course, all his doodads were on my uniform.

After this tumultuous beginning to my service in the Army, things settled down. I became good friends with a couple of my fellow Berry planners, one an aspiring pediatric cardiologist named Jim Kinney who wound up signing on for life in the Army Medical Corp where he eventually got a plum of a job at Madigan Army Hospital in Spokane, Washington. There he practiced pediatric cardiology, including holding a monthly clinic in Anchorage, Alaska, and retired as a Brigadier General with all the attendant benefits after 20 years of service. Jim and I used to run two miles every noon around the parade ground in the intense heat. When he was transferred to another Army base in Arizona, I discovered that he had kept all the scrubs that her wore for these runs in the trunk of his car until his departure.

I, on the other hand, despite promotion to Major and a Service Medal, resigned my commission at the end of two years' service determined not to have my career interrupted again. The medal was recommended by Dr. John Foley, my new Chief, for taking care of a handful of children with cancer with great difficulty and emotional cost as I was a true rookie in a very difficult area of medicine. I think this was the first time I ever lost a patient to cancer (leukemia) on my own watch without the support of a whole team.

Her name was Annette, about 5 years old which is typical. I was present when she died and sickened by the smell of blood since she essentially bled to death, painlessly, for lack of blood platelets to control the bleeding. I grieved with the family, developed an ulcer, and needed endoscopy for which I foolishly declined sedation. This was another first for me, unforgettable, for better or worse. I stayed in touch with the family, and the young mother developed early onset and ultimately fatal breast cancer within two years of Annette's death. We know now that she was at risk for this and might have prevented it by prophylactic intervention. I lost track of Rick, the father and husband. Perhaps he'll come across this book. I also lost a little boy with the same disease who used to call his penis his "dingdong" and a teenager with fulminant systemic lupus as well as a few newborns. These traumatic events helped prepare me for a future full of losses softened by rare triumphs.

Another Army experience of a lighter nature is worth reporting. One of my colleague pediatricians, Dr. David Tuberville, a good- natured young man, had just returned from leave. I noticed on the daily schedule that I was to see a family with several kids afflicted with lice. I asked for the children to be seen in Dr. Tuberville's room instead of my own. As I was examining them, Dr. Tuberville entered the room. Surprised to see me there, he asked why I was using his room. I responded, "These children have lice. I certainly don't want them in my office".

By the time I left Georgia for Los Angeles to continue my fellowship, I had gained a measure of appreciation for the South, its beauty, literature, and hospitality, and for the military where good people do good things under challenging circumstances. Despite my tendency toward rebelliousness, encouraged by my wife, Irene, I was still from a family that took its American citizenship very seriously, and I did too. As time has gone by, I have been moved by understanding that those that serve their country, not just in the military, are more likely to appreciate what they have and seek to improve it and own it.

I am proud now of my service, no matter how inconvenient. I am especially interested in the veterans whom I do not believe are sufficiently appreciated or reciprocated for their sacrifice. Many are minorities or other underprivileged people who gain confidence and respect through their service, but often fail to ever fit into civilian life where they are misunderstood or even maligned for doing what they believed to be their duty. We have served them poorly, especially with regard to PTSD and head injuries. There is now growing evidence that PTSD and head injury are closely linked. I can't help but think of Senator John McCain as I write this. I certainly didn't agree with him on most issues, but respected him enough to grieve deeply when he passed and left a huge vacuum of political Courage behind. I am now, aged 75, purely by happenstance, in a position to treat blast head injury and military PTSD with hyperbaric oxygen and conduct research to improve the marginal results. I will provide more details in a later chapter regarding this matter.

Today, I watched a compelling interview of a Congressman who was in charge of the Funeral Guard at Arlington National Cemetery, an elite organization of the brightest soldiers who compete to serve their fallen comrades by providing meaningful and perfectly executed farewells. These military funerals require disciplined soldiers, impeccably groomed, physically fit, composed at all times, and loyal to a cause in which they believe. I discovered the extent to which I have grown in my own appreciation of what the military does for us, and how far we have strayed from some of the principles that make them and us better.

I conclude this chapter by suggesting that non-compulsory, but highly attractive voluntary service to the country, following high school or GED, not restricted to the military, and rewarded by healthcare for life and at least partial funding for higher education, seems like a timely idea that perhaps one of the countless Democrats seeking the presidency might espouse as an unifying idea (imagine that). I still do not understand what has divided our country, but I am trying to gain some understanding of it which I believe is the necessary first step. Last year I campaigned on foot door-to-door for months in the midterm elections and was dismayed by the ignorance and apathy of younger voters, even in the era of Donald Trump.

This is how far I have come from my Yankee anti-military upbringing. One of my most meaningful personal relationships that I have had with a colleague in medical practice was with Major Wade Jensen, a military chaplain who served as Patient Care Coordinator in the brain tumor program at Swedish Hospital in Denver. I chose him for his sincere and shared belief that total care requires attention to the spiritual component of health. He and I remain categorically at odds over nearly every political issue, but remain bonded by our shared sense of duty, compassion, commitment, and mutual respect. He brought me a flag as a gift from his assignment in Iraq. I always opposed that ill-fated war, but the flag, a gift from someone who truly believed in something, is one of the few treasures which I kept close to my desk at work.

I hope this story has been of interest. Perhaps the lessons I needed to learn and did learn will have some positive influence in these difficult times. And so, with that notion, I am off to Los Angeles to continue my training.

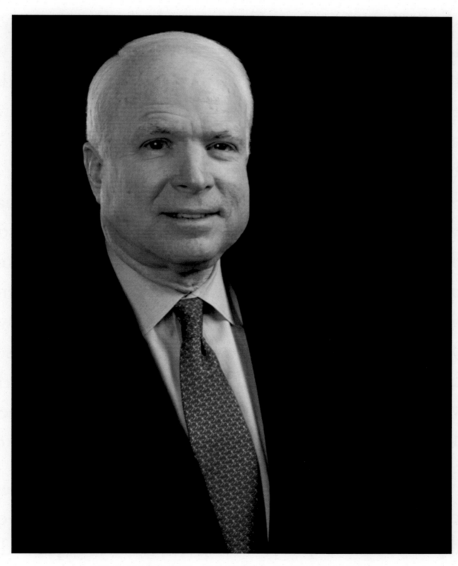

SENATOR JOHN MCCAIN
Published with permission of Arizona State University

CHAPTER 7

California Here I Come 1976-1982

My wife Irene, our two young children, Jennifer and Rebecca, and I departed from Fort Gordon, Georgia, which had recently built the much needed Eisenhauer Army Medical Center, after a very nice and emotional farewell gathering at a local watering hole. We headed toward Los Angeles, the questionably named City of Angels, where I would continue my training as a post-doctoral fellow at UCLA. I was to be mentored by Dr. Robert C. Seeger, an obsessive, and not clinically inclined researcher in tumor immunobiology, the field I had chosen for my research. While establishing my research, I would also continue part-time clinical work and some teaching of other fellows and medical students thus qualifying myself, if possible, as a classic academic "triple threat". Bob Seeger had been trained in immunology, (he was not an oncologist,) by Robert A. Good at the University of Minnesota, a true superstar known for his opportunistic interest in rare disorders of the immune system in children to better understand how the immune system works, something he termed "informative experiments of nature".

On the way from Georgia to L.A. we made a large diversion into central Michigan to see the vanishing Kirtland's warbler. Georgia had been a good place to develop my birding interest which proved crucial to my ability to continue my challenging work with childhood cancer. The trip to Michigan took us many miles out of our way, but we were able to bear witness to the preservation of a critically endangered species which had been saved through the teamwork of committed conservationists just as my colleagues and I were trying to save our patients.

The department of pediatric hematology/oncology at UCLA was led by a lovely man and excellent teacher, Stephen A. Feig, who had been trained under two towering figures in his chosen field at the Boston Children's Hospital, part of Harvard Medical School, Drs. Lewis K. Diamond and David Nathan.

Steve was and remains a brilliant man whose lab research was modest, but whose leadership, teaching, and clinical skills made up for it. He was also politically astute, but I always had the feeling that he did not want to see any of his protegees become successful enough to threaten his position; it never happened. He had a wonderful sense of humor which I hear myself alluding to often this many years later, black humor of course, necessary for finding humor in humorless situations to make them less intolerable. An example: the chemotherapy drug, BCNU is used mostly for brain tumors which are often fatal. After visiting a patient to whom we planned to give this agent, Dr. Feig said goodbye by saying "Be see'en you". Another example: A patient with a rare anemia called Blackfan-Diamond Syndrome after its descriptors was the child of an African-American and a Scandinavian. After seeing the patient, he waited until we were out of earshot and said that this version of the disease should be called the Black Finn-Diamond Syndrome. He also, quite correctly, alluded to the local architecture as "California Nouveau Gauche".

I began my research studies to prepare an experimental plan and quickly found myself so low in the pecking order that one of the research nurses entered a room where I was reviewing literature, looked around, said "I guess there's no one here" and left. With very little patient contact, I was clearly out of my element. I was also out of my element financially having left rural Georgia for La La Land. The price of rent was staggering and the price of buying was orders of magnitude above my salary which, in 1976 was about $25,000. Two years later, when I was "promoted" to the faculty as Assistant Professor, my salary escalated to $40,000. I should also mention that while I was training in Denver before my Army stint, I was paid an average of $9000 per year for about 70-80 hours of work per week and still had to pay taxes on it; I was below the minimum wage, even for that time, a clear case of discrimination against "soon-to-be-rich" MDs. The Army was a little better, and I was able to purchase a house to save on taxes, but that was Georgia. I was also confronted daily with the lack of the material things, especially cars, which seem so important to Californians and which is one of the reasons that the city still lacks a good public transportation system which could go a long way toward mitigating its smog problem.

I spent a couple of months at the library setting the stage for a quest to study a white blood cell called a macrophage and its potential to attack tumor cells. I joined the Senior Immunobiology Group which had weekly presentations by investigators and fellows, both MD and PhD mostly looking at the issue of the day, tumor immunobiology, in which it was believed that cancers grew only if they escaped the body's immune surveillance, and that if we could overcome this tolerance, we might find the cure. We submitted a multi-million- dollar research grant (Program Project) aimed at this subject from numerous directions, and my part was funded. This paid for my two years of research on the role of the macrophage in tumor control from which I published one important paper demonstrating that there are sub-populations of macrophages that do different things, previously unrecognized.

My paper was published in the prestigious Journal of Clinical Investigation for which I was called to the office of the Chief of Pediatrics who graciously commended my work and offered any assistance he could give. I told him that helping me buy a house, even if it were a large tent on Ballona Creek, L.A's concrete river, would be of great help. He did not see the intended humor, and no help was forthcoming.

Subsequently the macrophage world has evolved in a way that gives me some small satisfaction even though I did not stick with it for a number of reasons. These cells are used to make a few successful cancer vaccines and assist in producing a therapeutic immune response. We also know that there are inflammatory macrophages (type I) which respond to chronic inflammatory conditions including non-healing wounds, and other "healing" macrophages (type2) which produce growth factors that heal wounds or other inflammatory conditions. Ironically, it is a real possibility that, after all these years, I might have had an opportunity to enter into a collaboration to study how to classify non-healing wounds based on their population of macrophages and possibly find a way to coax the macrophages into the healing cells we need to close these refractory wounds.

I return briefly to the subject of using the immune system to fight cancer. Our initial efforts were largely unsuccessful because it turns out that cancer cells are so similar to normal cells that they usually don't elicit any meaningful immune attack. When the immune system, however, comes from a a donor who is not an identical twin, it is able to selectively recognize cancer cells, especially leukemic cells, and eradicate them in the context of bone marrow transplantation. While at UCLA from 1976 to 1982, I was an active participant in the fledgling bone marrow transplant program led by Dr. Robert Peter Gale. These were scary days. In fact, one of our chemotherapy regimens that we used to kill leukemic cells as well as the patient's own immune system to allow engraftment of the donor's bone marrow was eponymously called SCARY to signify the group of drugs used. Most patients suffered so much tissue damage beyond bone marrow that they never left the hospital and often died painfully.

However, those patients that survived seemed to be cured so that our task was to reduce toxicity. We had noticed that when we used identical twins for marrow donors, we never achieved cure, but when we used matched non-identical siblings or other family members we did achieve cures which were always attended by some manifestations of something called graft vs host disease (GVHD) in which the engrafted immune system attacks its new and foreign host, often with devastating consequences, but without which cure is not possible. Since then, we have been able to reduce toxicity of the preparative chemotherapy and/or radiotherapy regimens and focus more on management of GVHD. The results, as expected, have improved greatly. I was an author on the paper which convincingly presented the case for the "graft vs leukemia effect", its first description, which is now universally accepted. Unfortunately, this phenomenon seems to be restricted to leukemias and lymphomas and not the more common solid cancers. Our challenge is to find strategies to make these more common tumors equally amenable to immune attack from donors or from the patient's own immune system. I will return later to the issue of tumor immunobiology and its current status, but I would like to go back to my evolving career and other events of note at UCLA.

While struggling with my identity and my role at UCLA, I encountered a number of people who had an impact on my future career which, frankly, at this time was an enigma to me. Let me start with my research mentor, Robert Seeger. He was a friend, but worked so compulsively that someone might conclude that such behavior was necessary for success in research. If so, I was not interested. I had a life beyond medicine including family, running, and birding of which I have written my memoirs. Ultimately, Bob opined correctly that I was not sufficiently committed to research to be successful and harvested the remaining funds from my portion of our grant for his own work. I couldn't complain because he was correct.

Dr. Robert Peter Gale, Director of the Bone Marrow Transplant Program, who was brilliant, but quite arrogant and ruthless, encouraged me to "seize power" from Dr. Feig and become the leader of the children's transplant program. Lacking the desire for power and the obsession to acquire it, I did not pursue this and remained stagnant in the faculty academic ascendency game. Despite this, Bob Gale and I have maintained mutual respect, and later, after I had relocated to Albany Medical College, I got him invited to speak at the commencement of the Medical College about his efforts, supported by Armand Hammer, to travel to Russia after the Chernobyl disaster to attempt to do bone marrow rescue procedures on victims who would otherwise die of marrow failure. He had some success and good intentions which later included a failed attempt to get the Nobel Peace Prize. Nevertheless, his grandiosity was impressive and did involve Courage, a rare quality which comes up often in this memoir.

Other very notable personalities who graced the hallways of UCLA Center for Health Sciences in those days included Drs. David Golde, Martin Cline, Gerome Groopman, and Andy Saxon. Let me say a few words about each.

Drs. Golde and Cline worked together in the field of bone marrow culture and cloning of bone marrow growth factors. They co-wrote a tome on the white cell which was authoritative at the time. They were funny in a sarcastic way and headstrong at the pinnacle of their careers. Dave eventually left to head his department at Memorial Sloan-Kettering in New York where his depression eventually led to suicide, and Martin was caught circumventing UCLA's Human Protection Police by doing experiments in Israel that had been denied him in the U.S. He successfully implanted the gene for resistance to the chemotherapy drug methotrexate in human subjects, then subjected them to very high doses of the drug. It worked, but he got caught, lost his lifetime endowed professorship, and was exiled to private practice. He had always been a bit of a thorn in my side by insisting that my subpopulations of macrophages were nothing more than mature and immature versions of the same one-dimensional cell. He was wrong, but it stung.

Dr. Gerome Groopman, on the other hand, along with an immunologist named Andy Saxon, famous for overnight boat trips to the Channel Islands to catch spiny lobsters and driving an ancient car with a bumper sticker that said "eat my dust", were the real deal. Once it became clear in the early 80s that the AIDS epidemic was real, they played a major role in its diagnosis and treatment. Dr. Groopman is now well known and respected for his contributions to the compassionate and non-judgmental management and support of the tragic victims of this catastrophic infection. I am proud to have known him in his formative period which overlapped mine.

Despite the modest successes described above in research, I always felt that I was not a true triple threat and that my commitment to medicine, which arose from childhood experiences related in earlier chapters, was principally as a bedside clinician with knowledge of and great respect for clinically applicable research. In short, I was unhappy trying to create a fictitious persona. This discontent and my unhappiness with living in relative poverty in Los Angeles began to wear me down. I sought solace in long runs and birding. My wife was not interested in my career development or my melancholy, but was an outstanding mother of our two daughters. We grew apart, and I fell in love with a young nurse. I looked for a position in my chosen field in Calgary, Edmonton, and Hershey, Pennsylvania, but, in order to be closer to my children who had moved with my wife to Trumansburg, NY near Cornell University, my undergraduate alma mater, I accepted a position as Associate Professor and Section Head of Pediatric Hem/Oncology at the Albany Medical College.

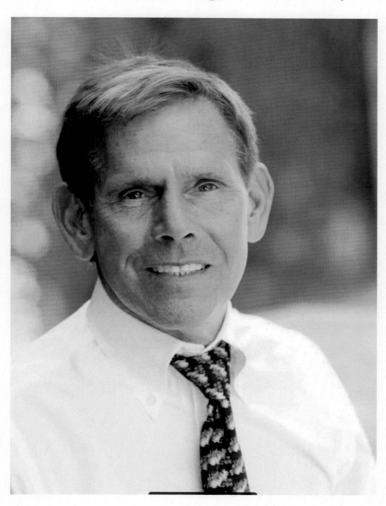

ROBERT PETER GALE MD
Obtained photo from Dr. Gale

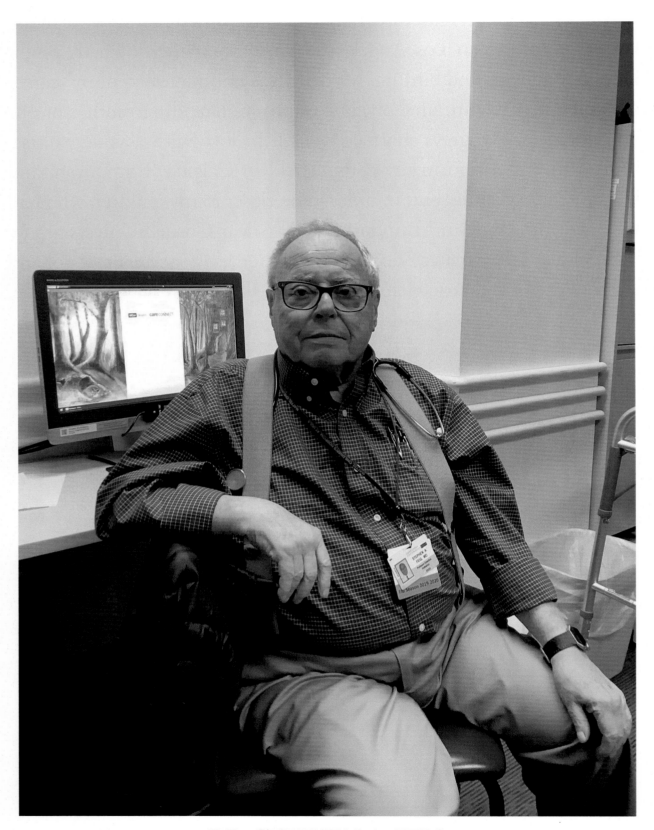

DR. STEPHEN A. FEIG
Photo provided by Dr. Feig, *Mensch 8*

Chapter 8

Back to New York: My Time as Section Head of Pediatric Hematology-Oncology at Albany Medical College (1982-88)

There my new boss was an immunologist who, like Bob Seeger, had trained with the legendary Robert A. Good (RAG). His name was Bernard Pollara MD PhD., a jolly, but intense Sicilian who said I looked like Jesus, (long hair, beard, and Jewish features,) and feared me. The program was marginal, but I was in charge and made it better by contributing to the formation of comprehensive programs for sickle cell anemia, hemophilia, and childhood cancer as an affiliate of UCLA in the international children's cancer research consortium known then as CCSG, Children's Cancer Study Group. This large group created clinical trials for most children with cancer along with a competing group called POG, Pediatric Oncology Group. I initiated a support group for parents, and hired a superb nurse practitioner, Megan McCabe, and a second oncologist, Dr. Jennifer Pearce from the University of Michigan.

While in Albany I was divorced from my first wife and married Julie Davis in 1984; We had two children, son Robin and daughter Patricia to add to the two I had with Irene. I was the only oncologist on the faculty and was therefore always on call. In order to visit my two older daughters, Jennifer and Rebecca, near Ithaca, I had a four hour twisty drive each way which I would do, round trip, in the same day stopping along the road at telephone booths to see if I had any calls; there were no cell phones in the early 80s. On Friday nights after work, many of the staff met for some carousing at the West End Tavern, purveyor of great pizza, greasy home fries, and Genesee Cream Ale on tap. I was careful to stay sober, but sometimes got a bit mischievous and called the on-call resident to warn him/her that, for example, a busload of hemophiliacs, all bleeding from an accident, were on their way to the ER or that a pregnant woman was coming in with a cobra bite. We did have some fun.

Let me start with Father Bentley and "his boys". Father Jim Bentley was the hospital chaplain in a predominantly Catholic town. This was years before the revelations of childhood sexual abuse by priests. He warmed quickly to the childhood cancer program and volunteered to spend time with the kids. It took me a while to realize that he volunteered exclusively with boys. We had a particularly difficult case of a teenaged girl with a fatal sarcoma who lived in a filthy tenement inhabited by variable people of questionable relation as well as a Noah's ark of stray animals and insects. The place was as foul and unhygienic as I have ever seen.

One night I got a call from hospice that she had passed away. I called the Father, and he agreed to make a joint house call to pronounce the patient and provide whatever comfort we could as well as Last Rites. He showed up, proved to be extraordinarily helpful, and I left with great gratitude. While we were there, I was horrified to watch cockroaches crawling on my patient's still warm, but dead body-a true defilement. When I returned to my apartment late at night, I shed all my clothes in the hall and went, butt naked, straight to the shower. Father Bentley was able to help me with this trauma (although the memory has never dimmed).

During my tenure in Albany, Father Bentley was suddenly transferred elsewhere and never returned. We were given no explanation nor his whereabouts. A few years later, I learned that his recreational activities with the boys were more than recreational, much to my shock and revulsion. I still cannot reconcile the guileless empathy that he demonstrated with his predatory behavior except to say that such men are not purely evil, but afflicted by something we simply do not understand. Of course, that does not excuse the Church's egregious handling of the matter, but perhaps does provide some insight into why leaders might have been as forgiving as they were notwithstanding the tragic mistake of failing to protect other children once the perpetrators were identified.

At that time, we had come to the realization that childhood leukemia, previously universally fatal, could be cured, but with quite toxic and occasionally fatal therapy including frequent spinal taps. The CCSG decided to do a randomized trial to see if we could achieve the same results with less aggressive therapy and obviate some of the risks. One of my patients, a bright 8yo girl, was assigned to the lighter arm of the trial. I adored this quiet, but sweet and affectionate child who was wise beyond her years, something that I have observed multiple times in children who inexplicably, seemed to be at higher risk for a bad outcome.

Unfortunately, she got the wrong therapy, and despite the good intentions, relapsed and became terminally ill. She accepted her fate, about which I was honest with her, with grace and never complained. When she was in her last hours, I came to the house and held her along with her parents and watched her leave this earth. There is no way to ever let this memory fade, but her peace gave me peace. I had to bear some responsibility for her failed therapy, but shared it with many others. The study was terminated, and we went on to refine, but not decrease the treatment for this most common of all childhood cancers.

Another patient with acute leukemia, Jimmie, had Down Syndrome which carries a higher risk of leukemia, but not necessarily a worse prognosis unless other serious manifestations of Down Syndrome interfered with proper treatment. He needed a bone marrow transplant, but lacked any full siblings, each of whom would have had a 25% chance of being a donor match. Instead we were fortunate to find that his maternal grandfather, who was in his 70s, was a match. We did the transplant at UCLA, and it was successful. I have lost track of him and his fiery single mother advocate, but stayed in touch long enough to know that he prospered as an unusually high functioning and charming Down Syndrome kid.

My relationship with his mother, a biochemist, was problematic; we had several serious arguments about his care which centered on poor or inconsistent nursing. She was a highly motivated and admirable advocate for her disabled child, but her sharp tongue and vigilance actually intimidated the nursing staff so much that many of the nurses asked to be excused from his care. She and I finally had a showdown in which I explained that she would have to make a choice between the marginal nursing staff with me as her son's oncologist, or be referred elsewhere for care. She and I finally reached a peaceful agreement that he was better off with me since I was fully committed to his care rather than take the risk of experiencing bias against her son somewhere else.

This unfortunate bias included my former mentor, Steven Feig at UCLA although the bone marrow transplant was done there. As a result of all this, I wrote a paper summarizing the results of all the known transplants with Down Syndrome which clearly showed that they did just as well as genetically normal children. I think this paper was influential enough to change many attitudes and allow more equitable care. Several months after the boy's transplant, his grandfather died, but remained mortal inside the body and bone marrow of his grandson. I have learned recently that this child remains alive along with his mother and his grandfather's bone marrow cells.

Occasionally in medicine, once you have established a trusting and open relationship with patient and parent, humorous things can occur. In the case of a young boy with childhood leukemia, things might have gotten out of hand and might have put me in jeopardy. Billy always approached his bimonthly spinal taps the same way. He held still, but generated considerable noise, and while I typically sang country folk songs for distraction and humor, he would loudly yell "take it out" over and over until the procedure ended. Of course, his mother was always encouraged to be in the room and was present one day when I asked her if Billy had learned this mantra from her. After a brief awkward silence, we all burst out in laughter except Billy who didn't understand the "joke". The laugher came as a great relief to me since I might have otherwise found myself in some difficulty. This episode, which under present circumstances might be a very serious problem, occurred spontaneously in the presence of a mother with whom I had a very good rapport and who I knew had a great sense of humor. The words just came out of my mouth under the stress of the moment. Political correctness certainly has its place, but sometimes it can inhibit doctor/patient interactions in a negative way.

Another story worth relating of my days in Albany is my relationship with Megan McCabe, my oncology pediatric nurse practitioner. She was petite, with dark hair and huge eyes, a real Irish beauty. We worked side-by-side daily and, although she was overly judgmental of various staff, I "nearly" always backed her up. I would say that she was occasionally flirtatious. When I arrived in Albany, I was separated from my first wife, but committed to my ultimate second wife, Julie, who was still at UCLA finishing her RN degree. I wore no ring, so I encountered several episodes of women who demonstrated "interest" in me. None of these episodes led to anything including Megan. The perception, of others, however, was somewhat different. I asked Megan to try to be more professional, but she was hands on, perhaps a little like Joe Biden; it was just her way. Finally, I had to counsel her, and she took it poorly, but got over it. Others were more aggressive. One medical student asked me to escort her to her graduation; another nurse proposed getting more personal. The pretty Chief Resident asked me to a concert. Another nurse got me into her apartment on some false pretense.

I cannot truthfully say that I wasn't tempted, but didn't waver. Ultimately, Megan fell in love with one of the pediatric residents and kept it a secret. She confessed to me very sweetly, and I gave my unsolicited consent. She has been happily married ever since and thus ended the rumors of our relationship.

This anecdote, certainly a common theme, of men in positions of authority succumbing to their temptations with attractive women and, in many cases, abusing that power is a serious matter that has recently escalated. It especially reflects poorly on service professionals. It is a very complex matter beyond the scope of this book except to say that it is an issue of great importance without which a full discussion of medical practice would be incomplete. There is a Jewish set of preferred behaviors called midot, (as opposed to mitzvot which are laws). One of these is giving the benefit of the doubt--easier said than done. However, spreading rumors of inappropriate behavior is potentially disastrous and should be avoided at all cost. The best practice is to avoid mixing affection, no matter how innocent, with professional conduct. Let me give you one great example:

Dr. Audrey Evans is a retired childhood cancer doctor who worked for decades with Dr. Giulio D'Angio who was one of the first childhood cancer radiation oncologists. (see Chapter 6) They were at Philadelphia Children's Hospital, part of the University of Pennsylvania. Their collegiality was never in question, and some speculated, but there was never a single moment, to my knowledge, when they were observed to be out of character. Finally, after their retirement, they announced their love and got married. This is a great tale of romance out of which a good movie could or should be made, but it could have turned out very differently if they hadn't been the consummate professionals that they were. As the book continues, I am certain that there will be more allusions to this type of issue, i.e. the real person vs the professional persona (Bill Cosby for example).

While in Albany, the Chernobyl nuclear disaster occurred, now seen in a terrifying series on HBO. My old colleague from UCLA, Dr. Robert Peter Gale (RPG), as I mentioned earlier, travelled at considerable personal risk and some gain as well with a medical team to the USSR to attempt to help those whose bone marrow had been destroyed by setting up a mobile bone marrow transplant unit. I convinced the graduating class of the Albany Medical College to invite him to be their commencement speaker. He showed up, unshaven, but in his personally monogrammed shirt, at about 6 a.m., shaved, had some coffee, gave a scintillating speech about conditions in the USSR and its medical chaos, rushed to the airport, and disappeared. I have kept in touch occasionally and did so recently to get his opinion on the television series on Chernobyl which I found compelling. I wanted his opinion, and he gave it in several pieces he had written.

Finally, I cannot depart from Albany without paying tribute and expressing my sadness to my many hemophiliac patients who were part of our comprehensive program. Virtually all of them were exposed to HIV which, at that time, we had no means of eliminating from their lifesaving blood products. To the best of my knowledge, most or all died; perhaps there were a few lucky exceptions. This was certainly a great tragedy, but one which might have had the Darwinian benefit of reducing very substantially the world's population of much suffering hemophiliacs, for better or worse.

Soon thereafter, with an offer in hand to establish a childhood neuro-oncology program at my old digs at the Denver Children's Hospital, I decided to resign. I felt I was leaving Albany in good hands and had little else to contribute. It was hard to leave the good friends I had made, but the Rockies beckoned. I called my chief, Ben Pollara, to inform him personally of my decision. He was emotional on the phone and made the usual offer to do anything he could to keep me, but couldn't come up with any specifics. Shortly thereafter, I met with Megan to say goodbye. She was quite distraught having never bonded with my successor, Dr. Pearce. She was very pregnant, but pledged to do her best to uphold our high standards of care in an otherwise mediocre place. This would turn out to be an impossible task, and she moved on to do pediatrics with her new husband, Ken Kroopnik, have children and a good and productive career which continues to this day.

While in Albany, I had developed a particular interest in pediatric brain tumors, the least successfully treated of all pediatric cancers. This was difficult because the pediatric neurosurgeon at AMC was one of a handful of neurosurgeons that I have known, (and I have known many neurosurgeons,) who lack the Courage (not the anatomy) to do the necessary risky operations. It has always been my preference to take on the more difficult medical challenges where there is much to gain and little to lose if one is willing to accept the possibility of failure.

Sadly, I have never seen Dr. Pollara since I left Albany although we had a few telephone conversations. He was a Damon Runyan character for whom I had developed a sincere affection, but we didn't become close because I never left off asking him for things he couldn't or wouldn't deliver. Let me give you one anecdote about Ben before I depart for Denver. There was a male nurse on the pediatric unit who fell far short of our standards and had a poor work ethic. Megan, as was her wont, caught him, for example, making up vital signs and charting them fraudulently. This was reported, but nothing was done. On one particularly egregious occasion of incompetence that put one of my patients at risk, I lost it and called him a "lazy scumbag", something I regret, but cannot say was inaccurate.

Within hours, I was, as expected, called into Ben's office. As I sheepishly walked in, he sat safely behind his desk with his strapped-on readers resting on the tip of his ruddy nose with a piece of paper in his hands and a very stern look on his face. I sat down and silently waited for my rebuke. Dr. Pollara looked at the paper, then looked at me, back and forth, then burst into a fit of uproarious laughter with tears running down his Sicilian nose. "Lazy scumbag, lazy scumbag, at least you didn't say douchebag!" he roared. He finally calmed down and said, "Maybe it's true, but you probably shouldn't say it in public". That was it; I was excused. His next call, no doubt, was to his bookie. Ben passed away recently in Florida. He was much beloved by many, myself included. During my years in Albany, I had gained some maturity, often through my own mistakes. I had arrived as a very young and inexperienced clinician and left a little wiser and a few years older.

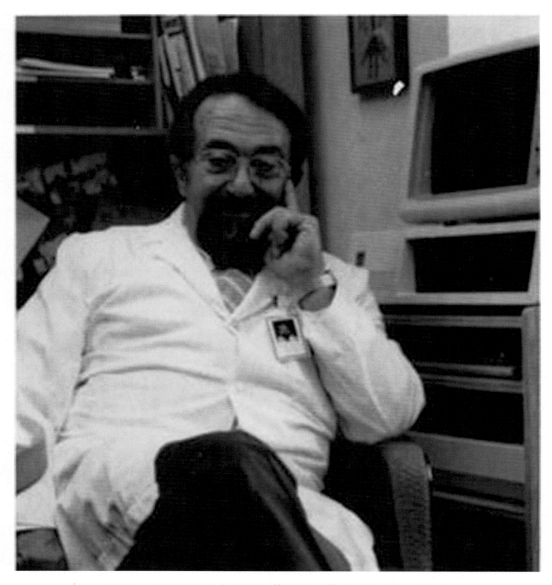

DR. BERNARD "BEN" POLLARA
Mensch 9
Photo obtained from Albany Medical College
with permission to publish

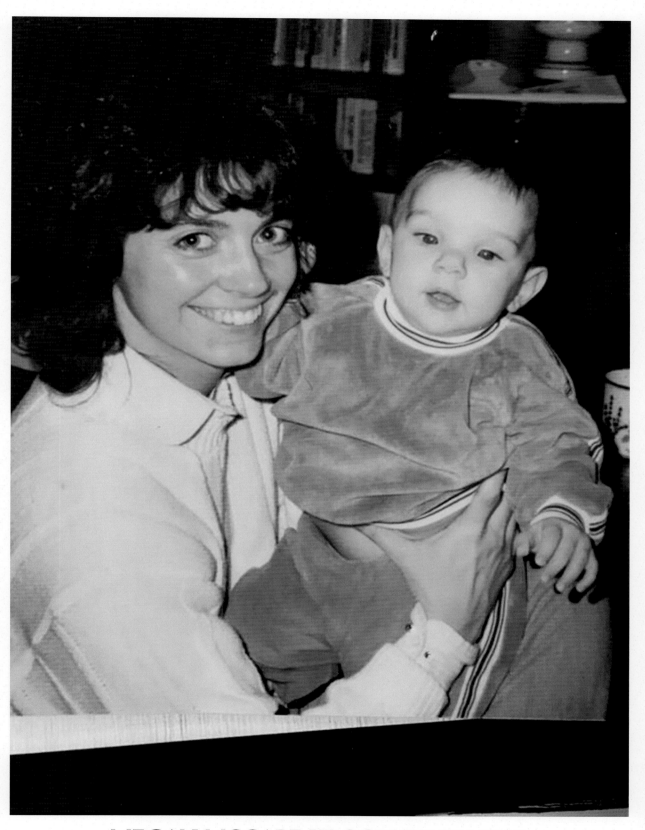

MEGAN MCCABE KROOPNIK RN PNP,
Mensch 10

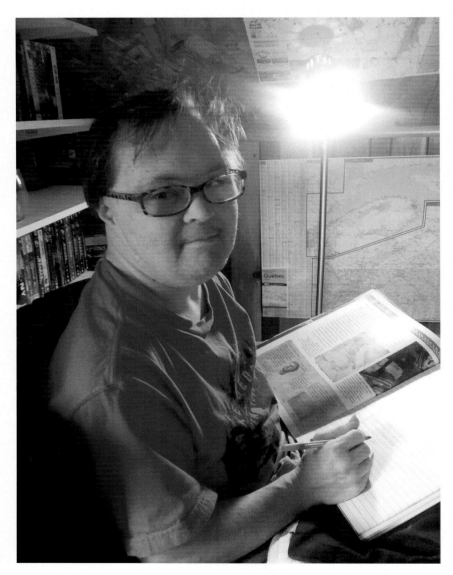

MICHAEL

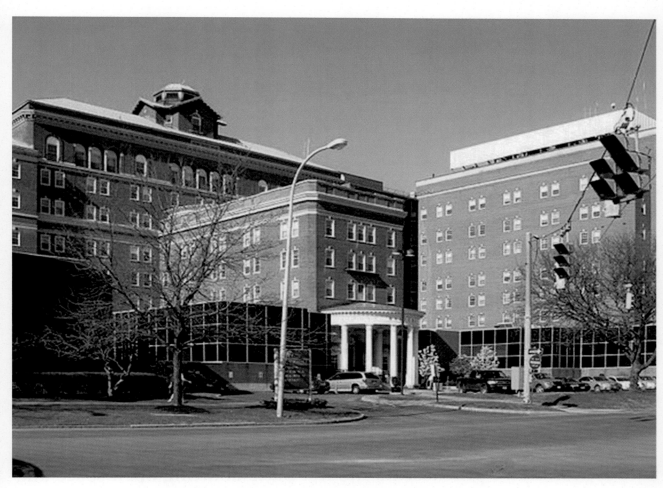

ALBANY MEDICAL COLLEGE

CHAPTER 9

Colorado Rocky Mountain High

Toward the end of 1987, my wife Julie, our son Robin, and my daughter Rebecca from my first marriage, who had decided to cast her lot with us, left Albany and headed for Denver. We found temporary lodging while we waited for the sale of our property in the Albany suburbs and acquired a knowledgeable realtor who showed us some developments which would allow access to Denver from the foothills of the Rockies. Some were picturesque mountain-view settings in the foothills west of Denver. We settled on a place called Ken-Caryl Valley which was a converted large ranch in the foothills with new model homes of various prices. We landed at 27 Buckthorn Drive which boasted horse stables, elementary schools just blocks away, recreational center, walking trails, open space, and strict covenants governing the pristine appearance of the Valley.

The original ranch house stood on a hill overlooking the whole fantasy world. We purchased a modest place abutting open space and moved in entranced by the beauty and wildlife. We quickly joined a "gourmet group" composed of anything but gourmets, but it gave us a quick social life. I had a considerable commute to Children's Hospital where I was happy to be re-united with some respected colleagues from the early 1970s. My daughter Rebecca entered Chatfield High where she excelled in track and cross-country and was homecoming queen. Julie became pregnant again and gave birth to my youngest, Patty, in 1989.

I assumed my role as oncologist committed to childhood brain tumors supported by a wonderful nurse, Gwen Mock, who soon moved to Minnesota where I have lost track of her. I found myself somewhat isolated from the other oncologists; they literally feared brain tumors. I was very busy with these patients and found little time for research even though I tried to establish a project with Dr. Ted Puck. He was a basic scientist exploring ways to achieve "reverse transformation" in which the malignant behavior of tumor cells might be reversed through chemical intervention. I discovered quickly that I could not make the required time commitment to bring this project to fruition even though I was aligned with an excellent young PhD candidate, Mary Haag. I was fortunate, however, to be able to teach some very bright young pediatricians who have become very successful, one was Jenny Kemp the daughter of our late former chief of pediatrics, C. Henry Kemp. Judy Bloomberg, now a superb pediatrician, was Jenny's alter ego. Another was Ken Cohen who later became a neuro-oncologist at Johns Hopkins. He and I saw eye to eye (nothing to do with my height).

In my efforts to expand upon the childhood neuro-oncology program, I partnered with a stellar neurosurgeon named Larry McCleary, well trained at Dartmouth College and Columbia University where he met his very eccentric wife. He was tied to the hospital, in all likelihood to avoid his wife's labile outbursts, and was often reported rocking his diminutive patients in the middle of the night. When he did go home to Genesee, west of Denver, he rode a Harley-Davidson *sans* helmet despite being well aware of the consequences of motorcycle head injuries. He routinely called me to the surgical suite when he was operating so I could see the tumor and learn the normal anatomy and help make some decisions. The situation was ideal, and we got off to a good start.

Radiation therapy (RT), while never something you would want to give to a child with a growing brain, was a staple and the main treatment available for treatment for those aggressive childhood brain tumors which could not be surgically controlled. The role of chemotherapy, pioneered by Dr. Victor Levin at UCSF, was just starting and unproven, but newer agents had become available to try, and some pediatric neuro-oncologists had attempted to use chemotherapy to avoid or delay RT, especially in infants. I joined this group philosophically and applied its principles to the treatment of all children with medulloblastoma, the most common malignant brain tumor of children the details of which are presented in the next chapter.

As is frequently the case, my initial enthusiasm for my new work environment was quickly abated for a number of reasons. One of my colleagues, a bright young woman from a pampered background made a point of doing things with her protegee which were helpful to her, but did nothing to enhance the reputation of the program. She, in my opinion, and as a member of the IRB which protected human subjects, violated its principals to skirt the rules, and I called her on it. I had proposed to our entire group that we help each other to be academically productive for the group benefit by sharing our clinical research, but she was not a team player.

The head of the department, Lorrie Odom, whom I had known for years, was not a strong leader and, although an excellent clinician, was not helpful in advancing the careers of her younger staff. She was not supportive of my efforts to establish some credible research, again in order to move forward academically. She was one of the old cadre of cancer docs with whom I had worked briefly before I left for my Army stint, and I did and still do owe her a debt of gratitude for helping us through those difficult days. I am still taking care of one of her patients, one of the first survivors of childhood leukemia, who now has late complications from the cranial radiation which helped cure her. I always contact Lorrie with reports on her beloved patient. I will return to this patient later in this work as she brings up some very important issues.

Another issue hanging over us as we toiled with sick children was the worrisome prospect of consolidating the Children's Hospital, which had always put patient care first, with the Medical School with which we shared staff and faculty, but had a much more research-oriented approach and clearly wanted complete control. Children's had been a place where community pediatricians could admit and care for their own patients with the aid of the house staff. Few of the full time Children's doctors were enthusiastic about this merger, and many of us formed a group self-named the Dinosaurs to meet and explore possible solutions. The inspirational leader of the Dinosaurs was Dr. Jack Chang, a superb pediatric surgeon, now deceased, about whom I would like now to spend a few more lines in tribute as I have in this book when the saga crosses paths with those people whom I have found most influential and inspirational; Jack was one of those *mensches.*

Mensch 11: Dr. Jack Chang

During my early pediatric training at Children's Hospital in Denver, Jack arrived from Duke University to practice pediatric surgery. He was 3 years my senior and ready for the limelight. Jack had emigrated from China with his family early in life to avoid communism and had become a star. He was always interested in liver surgery and eventually started the world's first pediatric liver transplant program while at U. Texas Southwestern in Dallas. He was a thinker and a Renaissance man who was an expert on whales and whaling history, but most of all a true gentleman. He preferred the clinical environment at Children's to the more academic, and perhaps more pretentious environment of the University Hospital as did I. One of his surgical sidekicks, Eli Wayne, who by Jack's standards was a bit rough around the edges, used to refer to Jack as the "Chinaman", the political incorrectness of which was so blatant that Jack actually seemed to enjoy it. Jack's surgical skills and keen intellect made him stand out, and I noticed.

When I returned to Children's in 1988 after being elsewhere since 1976, he was there as were several other familiar faces from the early days including Eli, Ed Orsini, Gale Levine, Lorrie Odom, and others. These formed the core of the Dinosaurs which eventually exited Children's en masse for the Rocky Mountain Hospital for Children at Presbyterian St.Lukes (PSL) Medical Center. This event was in response to the hostile takeover of Children's by the CU pediatric department. We all believed it would be the end of one Utopian place to practice pediatric medicine; it was. The new Children's, while certainly a fine place with millions of dollars in philanthropy, now resides in Aurora, CO near the old campus of Fitzsimmons Army Hospital, but its old identity as the home of the Denver pediatric community is gone forever.

Of course, Children's response to our move was hostile and dismissive. We were treated as if we were traitors. At a going away event, Chinese food was served, and I suggested that the host try her food before the rest of us ate; this did get a few laughs and broke the ice, but the ice was thick. The new enterprise which we launched in 1992, much credit to Jack Chang and his Courage, is still going strong and competes effectively with Children's which had to become monolithic to cope with the competition. The good news is that Camelot did not die, but simply morphed into a new program at a new location where the spirit lives on. Unfortunately, Jack does not.

He passed away from cancer in 2016. He was widely and deeply mourned, but he left a legacy of elegance in the practice of medicine that is unlikely to be surpassed. I would like to offer this anecdote to complete my tribute:

Once we were settled at PSL, I got to work with Jack more than I had before. When we had a new child with leukemia, for example, we would organize ourselves in the operating room so that we could non-traumatically obtain bone marrow, blood, spinal fluid, and place an indwelling catheter for non-traumatic venous access. Usually Jack, always the gentleman, allowed the oncologist, (me), to go first. One day we had such a case, and I had completed everything but the spinal tap. I had the area prepped and the needle in my hand when Jack broke his silence and said, "Did you ever go to Sturgis, SD for the big motorcycle rally?" I said to myself, this is strange, but answered "no" as we were not the biker types. He said "I saw a guy riding a Harley with a tee shirt that said IF YOU CAN READ THIS, THE BITCH FELL OFF". This was clearly calculated to disrupt what I was doing, and it worked. I laughed so long and hard at the utter inappropriateness of the joke, that I couldn't hold the needle still and had to delay the procedure for many minutes. I finally settled down, but it was a moment of collegiality, aimed to lighten a sad diagnosis, that I will always treasure. Of course, operating rooms are legendary for such occurrences, and that's where we were, in Jack's territorial comfort zone. Rest in peace, kind doctor. We all miss you.

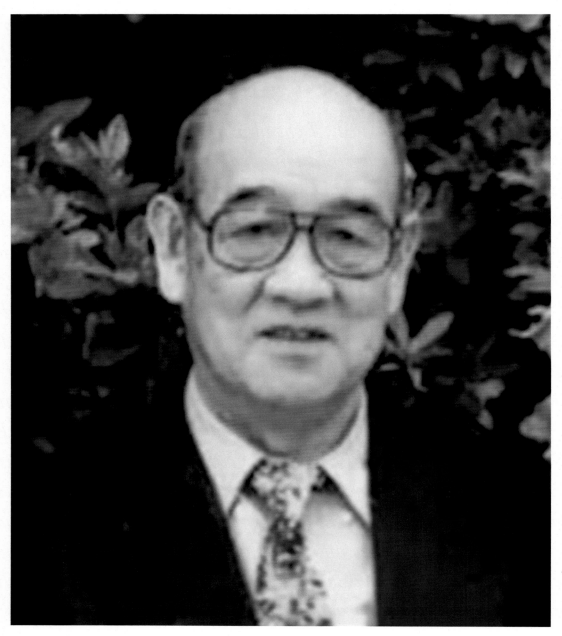

JACK CHANG MD
Photo kindly provided by family

At our new digs, John Cullen, Tom Smith, and I along with several superb pediatric oncology nurses including John's wife, Patsy, who is now at Regis University, formed one of the first ever private practices of pediatric hematology/oncology. We called it CHOA for Childhood Hematology Oncology Associates. We struggled to compete with our old department, but got by and delivered excellent care. This happened at a time when reimbursement for outpatient chemotherapy was high enough to cover the high overhead. Sadly, things changed because reimbursement was so poor and drugs so expensive that private practices could not make ends meet. Now there are very few really private practices anywhere that take care of cancer patients. Most oncologists who are not in academia work for large companies or hospitals where their freedom to practice the art of medicine is reduced to protocols and standards of care which are not always best for the patients. I will go more deeply into this timely and pervasive problem in another chapter.

CHAPTER 10

I End My Career In Pediatric Oncology and Begin My Career In Adult Neuro-Oncology, 1996-Present

After a few good years at CHOA, I began to see referrals of adults with brain cancer because of my uncommon interest in brain tumors and availability. This component of my practice become predominant, and the adults started to be uncomfortable in a childhood practice. Health One, a conglomerate of hospitals around Denver owned by a national corporation, HCA, formed and provided an opportunity to consolidate brain tumor services for the whole system. Dr. Michael Hitchcock, a neurosurgeon based at Swedish Hospital, and I hatched the idea of and attempted to set up regular conferences and form a team of doctors interested in brain tumors. Mike was affiliated with a non-profit called the Colorado Neurological Institute, based at Swedish, which could raise and allocate money to support clinical programs, education, and research in the various neurological diseases.

We very quickly learned that entrenched animosity and mistrust, some quite justifiable, made our original idea impracticable. We resolved to base the program at Swedish where it would be a new program of the CNI which we would co-lead. We created a brain tumor multidisciplinary conference which occurred twice monthly and was well attended by several neurosurgeons, neuro-psychologists, radiation oncologists, pathologists, neuro-radiologists, and others. At first, we actually invited the patients to hear our recommendations and ask questions, but the number of cases to be discussed grew and took away that option.

This conference began in 1996 and is now 23 years old and going strong. That means that we have discussed and formed care plans for about 6000 patients. As I facilitated these conferences, my goal was to emerge with a plan that everyone could support. Most of the time, we were successful. As expected, the cadre of neurosurgeons was the most likely to rebel. One in particular, a young buck, had an issue with the more elderly patients, regardless of their overall functionality, but kept his thoughts to himself unless I was not present. Then he would "go off" on me behind my back. Of course, this was always reported to me, and I confronted him until he finally backed off and ultimately migrated to Wisconsin. I have reserved an entire chapter just to deal with the potpourri of neurosurgeons with whom I have labored.

Once we determined to base our program, which we called the CNI Center for Brain and Spinal Tumors, at Swedish Hospital and CNI, we quickly built an unique program for patients which included coordinated clinical care anchored by a Patient Care Coordinator provided by CNI, a monthly support group, a monthly interfaith healing service co-led by me and the hospital chaplaincy, an annual celebration for brain tumor survivors, an annual memorial service, and an annual lectureship to which we invited many of the most prominent people related to neuro-oncology to speak to the professionals and to give another talk tailored to the patients and families to keep them informed. This list of speakers, to whom we gave an award for excellence, includes Dr. Mitchell Berger, Chief Neurosurgery UCSF, Dr. Raymond Sawaya, Senior Neurosurgeon MD Anderson Medical Center, Victor Levin MD, pioneer in use of chemotherapy in CNS tumors, Dr.

Linda Liang, UCLA neurosurgeon, Arie Perry MD neuro-pathologist, now chief of department at UCSF, Henry Friedman, neuro-oncologist Duke University, Paul Muller MD, Toronto, CA, Dr. Don Abrams Integrative Medicine SF, J. Gregory Cairncross MD, Canadian neuro-oncologist, Dr. Gregory Sorenson neuroradiologist, Harvard, the late Edward Oldfield MD, 1947-2017, NIH, and the late Dr. Judah Folkman, pediatric surgeon and visionary pioneer in the field of neo-angiogenesis. I will expand on this very worthy group and their individual and collective contributions with, of course, my personal reflections.

I think it is important to go into some detail about the interfaith healing service mentioned above. This was my idea, but strongly supported by the hospital chaplaincy. I believed that the optimum care of chronically ill patients should include attention to the spiritual needs of patient and family. At a time of great stress, especially with life-threatening illness, most people need and seek a connection with a higher power through some religious affiliation. Many are believers, but do not have a religious home, and even those who do have a place of worship often find little help there because it is disconnected from the rest of the care "team". We felt that by incorporating an opportunity for a spiritual experience into our multi-disciplinary program, we might provide better comfort and support. We created an interfaith service, co-led by me and a hospital chaplain, which acknowledged all faiths and pathways to spiritual connection and included music and poetry. The service was well attended and conducted in tandem with a support group facilitated by our patient care coordinator.

Patients and family members were active participants rather than just spectators. An article about this unique program was published in a psychology journal and discussed in the local news.

As expected, there were patients who actively avoided anything that evoked emotions that they feared and others who didn't attend because the service did not represent their personal beliefs. Most importantly, perhaps, was that the service provided me with an opportunity to reveal myself to my patients in a less clinical and more human setting where emotions were given permission to be expressed and where my staff and I often shed tears side-by-side with our patients. Every spring, we also held a memorial event for patients we had lost in which we lit candles for each patient, family members gave testimonials, and everyone shared in the sense of loss, but also in the hopefulness and renewal of spring. We planted an iris garden in which every flower represented a patient. This spiritual program is one of the innovations of which I am most proud and which I hope other programs will adopt.

I would also like to describe another part of our program that, subliminally perhaps, led to my later interest in the burgeoning field of cancer survivorship.

We held an annual event in the evening to celebrate our brain tumor survivors. We set standards of survival to qualify for this event so that patients would have some extra incentive which some clearly needed. For the more aggressive tumors, the cutoff was 3 years and 10 years for the lower grade tumors. We started in a private home with a handful of patients, then the program grew so much that we needed to rent a large space to accommodate about 200 people. We had not anticipated the great joy that this event provided to the survivors and their families to be able to share their good fortune with others in the same proverbial boat. We named each patient and their time since diagnosis, and each came forward to receive a candle which were all lit in unison to end the ceremony with, of course, a prayer. We provided an excellent meal and beverages with funds raised through CNI. Unfortunately, this and the Healing Service were among those components of the program that were lost when the hospital reduced and withdrew its support.

Let me provide further details of my personal approach to care of these adults with brain tumors. I decided, along with my superb nurse, Mary Pierick, who moved with me from children to adults, to continue those components of our approach to care which we thought were most valuable to children. Our rationale was simple: if it's good enough for children in distress, why shouldn't adults receive the same benefits? Mary, for example, was adamant and relentless in her determination to minimize any pain associated with treatment, especially unnecessary needle pokes. She terrorized the radiology techs by insisting that they leave in place the needles used to inject contrast material for the frequent MRI scans so she could use the same needle to obtain blood or to administer chemotherapy. I overheard a number of "conversations" that took place when the techs failed to comply with her "request".

For my part, I never wore a lab coat, never sat behind a desk, and always reviewed the crucial MRI scans with the patients and significant others in person on a large computer screen with the patient sitting on a comfortable bench facing the screen where I sat with my cursor. The MRIs were done and reviewed the same day to avoid even one sleepless night waiting for the life-or-death results. These sessions were conducted very informally, often with much humor when appropriate. In the case of either bad news or good news, I would summon Mary and the Patient Care Coordinator, (and my wife once she became my Practice Manager,) to share the experience with a prayer of gratitude for life and the moment. I established the practice, still in effect, of keeping an index of deceased patients organized by the month of their birthdays.

Each month, I sent the families a personalized card to acknowledge the mourned patient's calculated birthday and our continued concern. Needless to say, these were greatly appreciated and served to continue a relationship rather than allow it to end because we lost the patient.

My philosophy in building this program was to first establish a full service clinical program and team which included an approach to treatment based on what I had learned during my formative years in pediatric oncology which was essentially that our goal should always be cure and that, if we had that goal, we must take an aggressive approach to treatment which at least included a strategy for cure even though this goal might be elusive. At that time, we had not yet become enamored of newer treatments that are now used extensively as an addition to or substitute for conventional cyototoxic multi-agent chemotherapy. These include targeted molecular therapies and immune stimulators called check point inhibitors.

While the aforementioned novel treatments have added significantly to the cancer arsenal and have extended survival in several diseases, they are not curative, with the possible exception of melanoma which has always been an exception to everything. I have gone into great detail elsewhere in this saga about the development of multi-agent chemotherapy and the ultimate cure of most childhood and several adult tumors therefrom, so I won't repeat myself except to say that I made the decision early to apply this principle to the treatment of primary brain tumors in children and adults and have stayed the course ever since with considerable success.

Our brain tumor program began in 1996. At that time, a study had been published by Mark Gilbert and associates at the University of

Pittsburgh in which a combination of constant infusion cisplatin and BCNU, which required hospitalization, had produced very encouraging results in a small number of patients with glioblastoma multiforme (GBM), the most common and most lethal brain tumor of adults. Unfortunately, this regimen was quite toxic, and when an attempt was made to do a multi-institutional study with it, the original success could not be reproduced. I spoke to Mark about this at the time, and he indicated that the problem was unlikely to be that the regimen was ineffective; it was more likely that it was given by investigators who were not fully committed to risk-taking and therefore compromised the study by making unnecessary modifications.

I treated a handful of patients with this two- drug combination, and one is alive 23 years later albeit with severe peripheral nerve damage from cisplatin. Mark's observation was, no doubt, correct and unfortunately foreshadowed later events which negatively impacted the treatment of adult brain tumors. In the next chapter, I will present in detail my unique approach to the treatment of medulloblastoma, the most common malignant pediatric brain tumor and how it has influenced my approach to glioblastoma, the most common malignant brain tumor of adults

A final epitaph on the CNI Center for Brain and Spinal Tumors: The program was created in 1996, and in its prime, offered not only excellent coordinated multi-disciplinary clinical care, but also clinical trials, support group, monthly healing service, annual lectureship, annual memorial and celebration of life event, and more. By about 2010, Swedish Medical Center began reducing its support for the CNI, and these programs were all lost, one by one. You will not need me to tell you what the bottom line was that led to this unfortunate outcome.

While the program was being dismantled, the hospital was publicly reported to be one of the most profitable in the U.S.A. and its CEO was paid several million dollars per year. During this time, the hospital, apparently dissatisfied with its falling brain tumor market share undoubtedly caused by the dissolution and loss of dominance of its neurosurgical group, recruited a neurology trained neuro-oncologist, without any input from me, who arrived and promptly told all my referral sources that he was hired to replace me. A neurosurgeon was also recruited simultaneously who never referred a patient to me before he departed for another hospital. Nevertheless, I am still here as I write this, much to their chagrin, struggling to find suitable care for my numerous surviving brain tumor patients.

CHAPTER 11

The Sad Story of Glioblastoma (GBM), the Most Common Malignant Brain Tumor of Adults

During my years of practice in pediatric hematology-oncology, I recognized brain tumors as a major challenge in pediatric oncology. As has been my custom, I took this up as a special interest since there was a need, and most oncologists are particularly uncomfortable with anything that involves the brain.

The most common malignant pediatric brain tumor is medulloblastoma which occurs predominantly in the cerebellum, but also may occur less frequently in the cerebrum in which case it is called primitive neuro-ectodermal tumor (PNET). This disease, at least partially because it occurs in close proximity to the spinal fluid pathways, often spreads (about 30%) within the central nervous system to remote sites in the spinal cord and leptomeninges (membrane which surrounds brain and spinal cord). Its best treatment, following maximal surgical removal of primary tumor, is craniospinal radiation therapy (CSRT) in which the highest dose is given to the primary tumor (either just the tumor or the whole cerebellum) and a lower dose is given to the whole brain and spinal cord with great care not to miss any of it.

Craniospinal radiation (CSRT) is an effective and often curative therapy for patients with localized disease, but as we have learned, despite the adamant protests of a few, comes at a cost. CSRT damages the developing brain and impacts its maturation. It also affects other things such as spinal growth, thyroid and other pituitary functions, both central and peripheral, and exposes structures in the chest and abdomen potentially affecting intestinal function and the ability to tolerate chemotherapy.

Before the advent of effective chemotherapy, it was not unusual to find metastatic disease outside the central nervous system in bone, lungs, and other places including the peritoneal cavity, especially if a VP shunt was in place (a tube that connects the brain to the abdomen in order to drain excessive cerebrospinal fluid). Once effective chemotherapy was added, disease outside the central nervous system was essentially eliminated.

There was a particular reluctance to give full CSRT to very young children because of concern over their brain development, but this concern was perhaps misplaced since all children (and adults as well) were at risk for radiation damage which we know now is primarily based on small vessel vascular depletion which progresses over time as if it was a form of premature aging. Studies were conducted in which chemotherapy was given to at least delay if not eliminate radiation altogether. This included use of high dose methotrexate in an effort to manage disease which involved the spinal cord and /or leptomeninges. There was some success in this effort, mainly the recognition that medulloblastoma is a chemo-responsive disease in which chemotherapy might play various roles in gaining a better therapeutic strategy.

An approach which grew out of the effort to protect very young children was the notion that perhaps use of more aggressive chemotherapy might allow the dose of radiation to be lowered for all patients even if not eliminated. When I arrived at Children's Hospital in Denver in 1988, I was of the opinion that a more aggressive use of chemotherapy would be best tolerated if given before CSRT which significantly impairs bone marrow function and therefore tolerance of aggressive chemotherapy. I decided to treat newly diagnosed patients with localized disease in a pilot study the purpose of which was to maximize chemotherapy initially when it would be tolerated best and to delay CSRT, if possible, for one year. Then, perhaps, based on the observed efficacy of the drugs, the dose of CSRT could be lowered with impunity.

To do this, we used a combination of drugs, cyclophosphamide, etoposide, vincristine, and carboplatin which we called COPE. The regimen was given in doses calculated to require substantial hematologic support in the form of blood cell growth factors and transfusions and occasional admissions for fever and low white blood cell counts. This turned out to be the case, but careful monitoring and early intervention prevented any serious or life-threatening events.

We treated 11 patients with newly diagnosed localized medulloblastoma. All patients completed a year of primary COPE without tumor progression. At the end of a year, one patient refused radiation and ultimately relapsed and died. Another patient did get radiation, but had a late and prolonged relapse and died. The other nine patients, treated with 2400cGy of whole brain CSRT instead of the standard 3600cGy, but full dose to cerebellum (5400cGY), all survived. None demonstrated significant hearing loss from their carboplatin which, with standard therapy of cisplatin and higher dose RT, is nearly universal.

We presented these data in abstract form, but they were never published in a peer-reviewed journal since, when I left Children's Hospital, I did not get sufficient referrals of new patients to complete the trial. Furthermore, when I presented our data at a pediatric oncology meeting, I made the mistake of having two projectors as was fashionable, but experienced technical difficulties which gave me anxiety to the point of needing assistance to continue. I believe this created a distraction which compromised my presentation and its reception.

While the addition of chemotherapy in medulloblastoma has become standard, although not nearly as aggressive as what we gave, its use before RT has never caught on, and the dose of craniospinal RT has been lowered to 2400cGY. Additional decreases in the dose would certainly be beneficial, and the use of pre-RT aggressive chemotherapy provided the opportunity, but the necessary trials have not been done. This marked the beginning of a series of events for me in which creative and potentially important innovations were ignored for unclear reasons.

Subsequently, I have used the same approach in a cadre of young adults with medulloblastoma where outcomes are not as good as they are in children. The rationale was the same: use aggressive and effective chemotherapy, the toxicity of which is temporary, to allow reduction in the RT dose to the whole brain and spine. I have had only one death in at least 10 such patients. One, who had 2400cGy whole brain and spine RT, did have symptomatic chronic fatigue and evidence of microvascular injury which has been partially alleviated by hyperbaric oxygen therapy which I will discuss in detail in another chapter.

So, how does all this relate to the title of this chapter, The Sad Story of Glioblastoma? First, my approach of delaying definitive RT for children and adults was a radical idea at the time with which many caregivers, especially radiation oncologists, were not comfortable.

Second, the aggressiveness of the chemotherapy regimen, COPE, was more than most oncologists could stomach and required a good deal of time and effort beyond standard therapy. My background in bone marrow transplantation had prepared me to do this, but most of my colleagues were not similarly prepared. Finally, at the time that this pilot study was done, I was a member of the Brain Tumor Strategy Group for CCG, the Children's Cancer Group, which then merged under government pressure with the Pediatric Oncology Group to form the new Children's Oncology Group, COG. I attended the first brain tumor session of this group, and it was immediately obvious that I was being replaced and would have no influence. Those who were more recognized for their work in childhood brain tumors, mostly well-deserved, were not inclined to cede their positions of power and influence to a relatively unknown such as myself, and I lacked the ambition to fight.

This was a big mistake since I believe that I had ideas worth pursuing and was more creative and certainly more of a risk-taker than those in more influential positions. Possibly, in my current state of mind, I would have made the effort, but for personal reasons, I wasn't prepared for the struggle, avoided celebrity and its inherent obligations like the plague, and essentially dropped out. This was also the time that I made a switch from childhood cancer to adult neuro-oncology. Let me take some of your time to tell this story.

After leaving Children's Hospital to form a private practice of pediatric hematology-oncology in 1992, I started getting referrals, mostly from neurosurgeons, who were looking for someone with neuro-oncology expertise to whom they could refer patients after surgery and expect good care. This was new to me since in a children's hospital such referrals were not possible. At the same time, my pediatric referrals dropped precipitously since very few children had neurosurgery anywhere other than Children's. I accepted these adults and quickly realized that I had something to contribute. This was not necessarily well accepted by my adult oncology colleagues who had enthusiastically helped us start our practice. I was perceived as taking their patients even though they had no particular interest or expertise in brain tumor care. Furthermore, as a pediatric oncologist I was not viewed as necessarily competent to care for adults (a preposterous assumption as children are typically much more challenging). A meeting was called in which I was threatened with a plan to stain my reputation and make drug purchases less affordable, but I ignored the threats and continued with the adults. In the process, some bridges were burned, but "I didn't start the fire" (Billy Joel).

Once I found myself with the daunting task of managing adult brain tumors, the vast majority of which were glioblastomas (GBM), a highly malignant and "incurable" tumor, I had to decide how to treat them. At the time, surgery and radiation were the standard care with the option to use chemotherapy in the form of BCNU, a nitrosourea alkylating agent which kills tumor cells by irreversibly binding to tumor cell DNA and preventing cell division. This drug improved survival, but fell just below statistical significance.

The neuro-oncology group at the University of Pittsburgh had reported very encouraging results using a combination of infused cisplatin and BCNU over 72 hours in the hospital. I contacted one of the authors, Dr. Mark Gilbert, who encouraged me to try it which I did. It was quite toxic and the hospitalization was unfortunate, but I believe it was effective. My longest GBM survivor, now at 23 years, got this regimen.

Soon thereafter, however, a multi-institutional study led by Dr. Gilbert failed to confirm the benefit of this regimen, probably because of poor physician compliance. Dr. Gilbert agreed with my concern, but the data dictated that we discontinue this approach. This was just about the time that the drug, temozolomide (TMZ), an oral and relatively non-toxic alkylating agent known to cross the "blood/brain barrier", was shown in early studies to be effective in relapsed GBM. In addition, irinotecan, a drug which also interferes with tumor cell division by altering DNA, showed promise in early studies. I decided to create a 3- drug regimen which I called BITE composed of BCNU (B), irinotecan (I), and TMZ (TE) which would be given as often as blood counts allowed, every 4-6 weeks. We also initially included the drug Taxol, but dropped it because of excessive toxicity and because pending studies concluded that it was not effective in GBM. We would try to maintain dose and schedule in order to be as aggressive as possible and avoid the pitfall of the cisplatin/BCNU experience. We would give everything as an outpatient, but the BCNU would be given over 4 hours three days running to simulate the constant infusion concept. This approach was consistent with the "intent to cure" approach of using multi-agent therapy which was extensively discussed earlier with regard to the cure of childhood leukemia and Wilms tumor.

We launched this pilot study with IRB approval in 1998. We treated 35 patients, but the study was stopped because of a patient death associated with re-activation of a ubiquitous, but potentially virulent virus, cytomegalovirus. Subsequently, we have monitored for this virus and the immune system in general and have been able to avoid any more cases of this or other fatal opportunistic infections.

Once the study was stopped, we continued to monitor the treated patients and discovered an overall survival rate which was better than expected and justified an attempt to modify the regimen to make it safer and maintain its efficacy. We decided to only give BCNU after radiation therapy (RT) and only every third course in which we would substitute it for the irinotecan. All courses included standard TMZ which was given for 5 days monthly and daily during RT along with weekly infusions of irinotecan, but we were relentless in our zeal not to dilute the regimen with impulsive dose reductions. This approach turned out to be much less toxic, and we treated an additional 75 newly diagnosed patients with the modified version of BITE (mBITE).

As it turned out, our 75 patients were treated more or less simultaneously with over 300 patients on Dr. Roger Stupp's seminal study comparing RT plus TMZ to RT alone. This ultimately allowed us to compare our results to a simultaneous, but separate study of TMZ as a single agent compared to our 3- drug regimen. The results, all very statistically significant, showed double the overall survival for our patients compared to Stupp's at 2, 3, 4, and 5 years. Median survival was 20 months compared to 14.2 months with TMZ alone. Further, a subgroup of patients defined as more favorable based on age less than 60, good functional status, and gross total tumor removal at diagnosis was found to have a median survival of 36 months and a 50% chance of living 5 years. I submitted these exciting data in abstract form to the International Society of Neuro-Oncology Meeting to be held in Edinburgh, Scotland in the spring of 2010. With long follow-up, the results were particularly compelling. I expected to give a platform talk and thought it might be chosen for a plenary session. Things worked out very differently.

My abstract was chosen only for poster presentation, and no one showed up to discuss the poster. Later, I contacted Mark Gilbert to get his advice and found him cold and distant (and probably guilty).

He indicated that we didn't have enough molecular information to be certain that we had not treated a select group with a more favorable prognosis. Of course, Stupp's study had some data on this, but they did not correlate their molecular analysis with their outcomes, and only about 30% of patients had the favorable molecular characteristics.

As it turns out, only about 33% of patients in several studies have favorable low levels of MGMT, an enzyme which when present in tumor cells degrades the response to TMZ. This fact is part of the rationale for giving a multi-drug regimen which is what we did in order to compensate for the variable response to single agent TMZ. This is the same rationale that led to the cure of most childhood and several adult cancers, but had been forgotten in the case of GBM (or never known since most neuro-oncologists are neurologists whose training would not have taught them the lessons we learned in the 70s).

I was devastated by the snub of being relegated to the far corner of a huge room full of posters so that virtually no one noticed it. I had travelled all the way to Edinburgh believing that I had come across something worth fighting for and had been ignored. Subsequently, attempts to publish our data failed. We were told that we did not have a control group and that the data were therefore not persuasive. Our intention had been to round up other investigators to do a randomized trial (our program was too small) comparing single agent TMZ to mBITE, but that never materialized. Why?

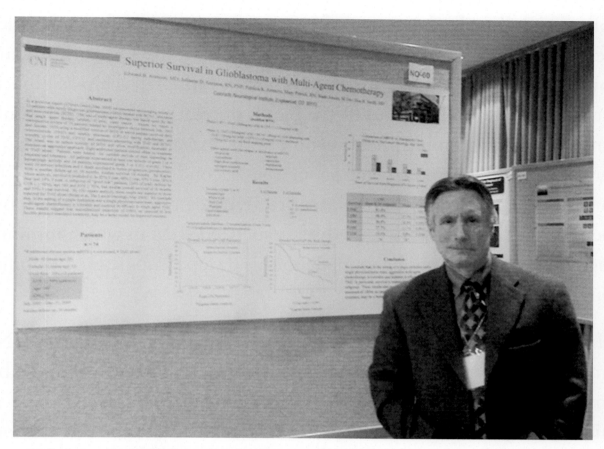

YOUR AUTHOR KEEPING HIS POSTER COMPANY

Well, I am not sure that I can answer that question to anyone's satisfaction, especially my own. Here is what I can say: despite the validity of the lack of MGMT analysis of my patients, the results were so superior to those obtained with "standard therapy", that at least they should have been presented in a forum where concerns could be addressed. Otherwise, there was the possibility, which turned out to be the outcome, that a far superior treatment for a fatal disease would be permanently overlooked; this came to be and remains the case.

Since then, I have continued to treat my patients with mBITE in spite of constant opposition from insurance companies and professional skepticism. As a result, I have a cadre of long -term survivors which predictably shocks my colleagues from prestigious institutions. The NCCN, (National Comprehensive Cancer Network,) a board of professionals involved in care of cancer patients, was formed which offers recommendations for treatment of all cancers. Once this board provided its "guidelines", insurance companies adopted them as Biblical truths which allowed them to tie the hands of creative providers. I would compare this predictable phenomenon to the extraordinarily damaging literal and Biblical interpretation of the Second Amendment to the Constitution. Of course, sometimes creativity can get out of hand, but when we are dealing with a fatal disease such as GBM in which minimal progress toward cure has been made to this day, perhaps some flexibility would be a wiser approach.

I have made several attempts to contact members of the NCCN's committee on brain tumors with no success. I have had innumerable conversations with physicians who represent insurance companies in which the physician clearly believed our data and understood my reasons for wanting to deviate from the NCCN standard, but who informed me that they lacked the authority to make an exception in the absence of a peer-reviewed article attesting to the value of my therapy. Unfortunately, my attempts to publish my results had been "unsuccessful".

At present, we are in an era of cancer treatment in which cytotoxic chemotherapy has been de-emphasized so that very few new agents are available for testing. An array of high tech. treatments such as molecular targeted therapies, immunotherapy, viral therapy, radio wave therapy, and many others have dominated the research scene. There has been progress from these approaches, especially in melanoma, lung cancer, kidney cancer, chronic myelocytic leukemia (CML), and childhood leukemia, but, with the possible exception of CML and rarely melanoma, no cures. In addition, these newer treatments are every bit as toxic as conventional cytotoxic chemotherapy, but their side effects are different and often more difficult to manage. Finally, by and large, these newer remedies are enormously expensive such that the ratio of cost to palliation of symptoms is often narrow, and none, with the notable exception of the anti-angiogenesis drug, bevacizumab, has had any efficacy in GBM.

So, here is where we stand in the treatment of GBM, a disease which afflicts at least 15,000 patients per year who are often in the most productive years of their lives. These patients, approximately 66% of whom have tumors that by virtue of their content of MGMT are relatively insensitive to TMZ, nevertheless get only TMZ in addition to surgery and radiation. Combination chemotherapy, the only known way to cure any cancer, is not recommended by the NCCN and therefore seldom given (a recent paper has indicted possible superiority of adding CCNU to TMZ, but has not become the standard). Even patients who are responding well to TMZ often have the drug arbitrarily and unnecessarily stopped prematurely because no studies have been done to determine the optimum length of treatment.

At the time of inevitable and predictable tumor progression, GBM patients are frequently put on phase I clinical trials which have a dismal track record for being efficacious. This is done in spite of the availability of bevacizumab (Avastin), a drug that inhibits production of new blood vessels and damages those that are already present. This drug is approved and effective for palliation in recurrent GBM, and in my experience, occasionally leads to long-term survival. Other cytotoxic chemotherapy drugs, such as CCNU and irinotecan, are also seldom given despite proven benefit in GBM. All this has led to a sobering lack of progress and, as we have seen in some familiar and beloved public figures such as Senators John McCain and Edward Kennedy and the son of Joe Biden, early demise, much to the detriment of our society.

Even lung cancer, a much more common disease with a dismal track record for survival, has far exceeded the progress made in treatment of GBM. In the context of what I have already said, the final factor to be discussed is how physicians approach patients with GBM. To make a long story shorter, there is a tendency for neuro-oncologists to become nearly robotic in their approach with a conspicuous nihilism and dependency on "guidelines" and corporate restrictions to guide their approach. Most work for hospitals or corporations such as Kaiser -Permanente or U.S. Oncology which are risk-averse and literally tell their physician employees how to treat their patients or face the consequences ($$$).

Coming from my early background in which risk-taking and creativity were all we could do and were only discouraged when we exceeded reason, these restrictions are abhorrent to me. I am fortunate to be at a point in my career when I can make the decision, albeit reluctantly, to retire with the knowledge that I have tried hard and, for the most part, done my best. The grief with which my patients and I are now processing our imminent separation is a testimony to the success of my now nearly extinct approach. Furthermore, the longitudinal care of adult brain tumor patients has been passed to neurologists, not oncologists, who have never experienced or been taught the principles of cancer care and especially intent to cure. This occurred to a great extent because oncologists abdicated their role to the neurologists for reasons that I could speculate about, but won't. In my own case, I plead guilty to the avoidance of celebrity and the cut-throat politics of medicine which led to less notoriety and fewer publications. Perhaps I should have been more aggressive, but then it wouldn't have been me.

Neurologists, no matter how bright and knowledgeable, are, with few exceptions, not cancer doctors, so it should be no surprise that they have taken, for the most part, the more comfortable approach of giving standard palliative therapy, then doing clinical trials, often phase I, the vast majority of which have produced negative results. We are really no better off in our outcomes for GBM than we were in the late 80s and early 90s despite an exponential increase in our understanding of the nature of cancer. It is a sad story, but one that needs telling. I take no pleasure in its telling other than knowing that it has been told and that some good might come from that.

CHAPTER 12

Mensch 12: Jay Schneiders, PhD, Neuro-Psychologist

When the Center for Brain and Spinal Tumors (CNI) was created in 1996, we had the good fortune to include Dr. Jay Schneiders, a PhD neuro-psychologist who was working with the epilepsy surgery program as well as movement disorders and any other neurological condition in which his services were required. A neuro-psychologist is trained to assist in the care of patients with neurological diseases. Their role is to assist neurologists, neurosurgeons, and, in my case, neuro-oncologists to better understand the functional consequences of neurological disease. They generally do not treat patients with primary psychiatric illness or do long term counseling although they are qualified to do so.

Jay was trained at Michigan State University and Brandeis College. He and his family had been very actively involved in the civil rights movement of the 60s. He is a published poet as well and a knowledgeable and practicing Jew. He and I bonded quickly as he proved to be extraordinarily "useful" in our developing program in which he was able to guide us in determining the initial neuro-cognitive status of our patients and assessing the consequences of surgery and other therapies needed to treat the disease. He was often present during surgery when patients were awakened during the operation to test their neurological status. He was not only highly knowledgeable, but compassionate and insightful about the various issues of life that might confound a good assessment of neurological status. Most importantly, he was not one to pontificate and disappear as I had encountered previously in my days at Children's Hospital. Instead, he was willing and able to be present at the most challenging times to assist in any way he could. This was also true of myself so that we often would work as a team in difficult circumstances. Let me give you an example.

Early in the Program, we had an unusual patient, a lovely African-American man who had converted to Judaism to marry his white Jewish wife. Unfortunately, he had a very large glioblastoma, the most malignant adult brain tumor, in a difficult location which made the surgery very risky. He was operated on by one of our younger and more talented neurosurgeons. Tragically, this patient did not wake up from his surgery and suffered massive swelling which precluded any chance for meaningful survival. Both Jay and I saw the patient and extended family the morning after the surgery which happened to be a Saturday, the Jewish sabbath, which both of us observe. I contacted the neurosurgeon for his input since we had to make some difficult decisions. He told me, quite briefly, that he was sorry about the outcome, but was not on call and would not be in to see the family. He supported any decision the family made and affirmed the extremely poor prognosis. So, it was up to Jay and me, although we hardly knew the family, to help them make decisions and support them.

Rabbi Bruce Dollin stopped by after morning services to offer his prayers, but could not do much else. He read some psalms and some blessings and departed. By that time, after hours of discussion involving the spouse as well as numerous friends and family members, (Yiddish term mishpucha,) we had made the decision to discontinue life support, but wanted it to happen after the sabbath (shabbat) at which time we would have a brief service which ends shabbat called havdallah. Rabbi Dollin had agreed to come in and officiate.

Jay and I went home for a few hours to get a little rest, then returned at sundown which ends shabbat. We all gathered around the bed in the intensive care unit, conducted the beautiful service, then stayed while life support and life itself ended. It was approximately 8PM; we had arrived that day at 8AM. It was a long day, but sad as we were, we knew we had done something special, and that we had helped each other get through it. This is, in fact, the best way that people who are in this challenging field can do what they do and keep doing it, by supporting and caring for one another. Unfortunately, the neurosurgeon was not there; he would have learned something that he probably still hasn't learned. Jay and I still talk about that life-changing day.

On a much lighter note, Jay has a wonderful and appropriately dark sense of humor for doing the work he does. I find humor indispensable. We frequently have lunch together in the doctor's lounge where we have been fortunate to be joined by a cast of characters that contributed much to humor that often escalated into laughter loud enough to get the attention of the many dour physicians in the room. These included Drs. Nathan Persoff, a recently retired superb family physician, Mark Kramer, a brilliant neurologist and epileptologist, Allen Bowling a neurologist who specializes in MS, and several others.

Most, but not all, were Jewish, but all understood and actively participated in our humorous escapades, many too dark to be reported here. In retrospect, Jay and I agree that these sessions were crucial to our success working together over the years. We still look for each other any time we enter the room and are disappointed if the other is absent. We have both gone through a number of personal crises since we first met, and we always have been willing and able to help the other without judgment. The take home message here is that the best friends are the ones who show up when things are the worst. They are few and far between, but thankfully that has been enough. Of course, we had a few disagreements along the way. These are unavoidable, but less painful when there is a meaningful relationship and mutual respect.

Jay has also recently assisted me in assessing patients before and after hyperbaric oxygen therapy and has bailed me out a few times with patients with severe needle phobias which he has skillfully solved in literally minutes much to the patient's (and my) benefit.

All I have said clearly qualifies Jay as one of the few associates who qualify in flying colors for classification as one of those menches whom I have known and whom I have chosen for tribute in this memoir. I was recently fortunate enough to employ his very beautiful and talented spouse, Anita, to help my wife and me sell our house, a very painful experience, which she, predictably, helped make tolerable and successful.

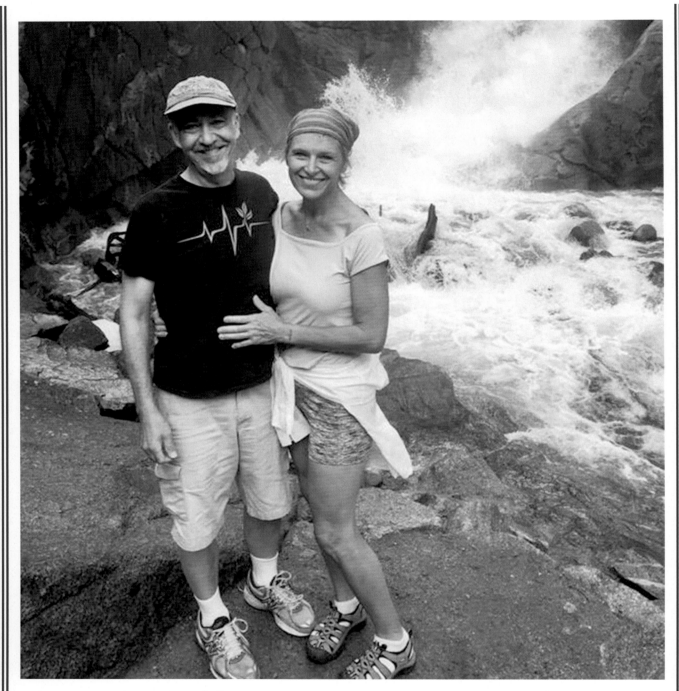

DR. JAY SCHNEIDERS AND SPOUSE ANITA

CHAPTER 13

Mensch 13: Mitchell Berger MD, Chief, Department of Neurosurgery, UCSF Medical Center

I have known Mitch for at least 30 years through my work in the Children's Cancer Study Group (CCSG) and as a colleague who has helped me with numerous patients over the years with almost universal benefit. He is a large, very approachable man who played briefly for the Chicago Bears after he was graduated from Harvard College. Of all the neurosurgeons with whom I have worked, and despite his very hectic schedule, he uniquely responds promptly to requests for his opinion and makes himself available at crazy hours.

Dr. Berger has pioneered the use of pre-operative and intra-operative functional brain mapping, often with the patient awake, in order to optimize tumor removal with preservation of function. He has published data clearly demonstrating the prognostic importance of achieving maximum tumor removal. If post-surgical therapy were more effective, surgery might not be as crucial, but very little progress has been made, despite a variety of new and exciting treatments for cancer in general so surgery remains, in my opinion, the most important component of treatment.

What this means for patients with malignant primary brain tumors is disturbing. If they do not have the good fortune to be in the right place at the right time, or if they are not referred to the right place, they are likely to have a substantial reduction in their chances for both survival and quality of survival. In a perfect world, all patients who have primary brain tumors would be referred to a handful of centers where the best neurosurgeons practice. It has been shown that volume does count; that is, the more brain tumor operations a neurosurgeon does, the better the outcome. Neurosurgeons are a proud, (and often cantankerous lot,) as they should be, but the pride that comes from rigorous years of training, can and does create a great reluctance to admit that there might be a better surgeon for a given patient; referrals are the exception, not the rule. The results speak for themselves.

Furthermore, the environment in which a neurosurgeon functions is likely to influence the degree of risk which that surgeon can tolerate. Alex West, a talented neurosurgeon who has been in both high academia as well as private practice, once told me that if he were in a place of higher prestige, and thereby protected from criticism, he would do more aggressive, (and appropriate,) operations on brain tumor patients. This candid statement was unexpected, but certainly true. The solution is elusive. I, however, at the risk of jeopardizing my own professional relationships and therefore my livelihood, have referred numerous patients, always to Mitch Berger, not because other neurosurgeons could not do the operation, but because Mitch is consistent, accessible, and his judgment is impeccable. I have had disgruntled neurosurgeons as a result of these referrals but, for the most part, they don't complain because they are not diminished in any way, and they know that he will do what they wouldn't; otherwise, referral would not have been necessary. As for those who did change their referral pattern as a result, to my detriment, I will let you be the judge.

I must, with reluctance, also say that many of the best neurosurgeons are to be found in centers with mediocre to poor neuro-oncologists. The neurosureons do their magic, then must watch as the patients are given *post-surgical treatment lacking in optimism, creativity, and even compassion. They are often channeled into clinical trials with little or no chance to be successful under the misguided philosophy that there is no better option. Much more about this elsewhere. As for Dr. Berger, he works with other professionals who are committed to the best possible care of their patients. But, unlike some other neurosurgeons, he always sends the patients back to their referring physicians without any poisoning of the water.*

As I write this, I am looking forward to visiting Mitch Berger and his team in September, 2019, to talk about the benefit of hyperbaric oxygen therapy for the treatment of brain tumor survivors who have been harmed by the late effects of their radiation therapy. As I approach retirement, I value this opportunity to express my gratitude for the role that Mitch has played in my career and the good that he has done for many of my patients and innumerable others.

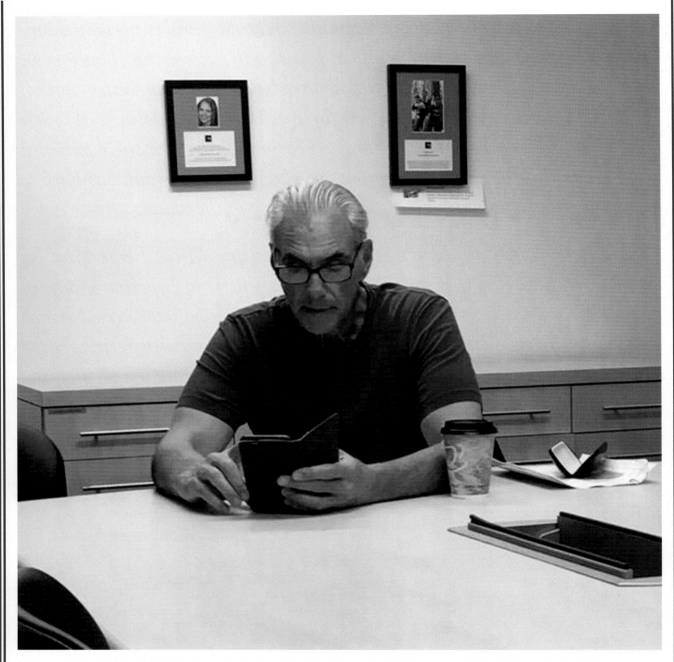

MITCHELL BERGER MD, CHIEF DEPARTMENT
OF NEUROSURGERY, UCSF

CHAPTER 14

Mensch 14: Judah Folkman MD 1933-2008

I had the good fortune to meet Judah twice. I first saw him in 1973 during my initial year of fellowship training in pediatric hematology/oncology at the Children's Hospital in Denver where he had been invited to give a talk on his research by his trainee in pediatric surgery, Dr. John Burrington.

His talk dealt with the topic of the requirement of tumors to make their own blood supply to grow beyond a very small size, perhaps 4mm. It sounded interesting, but not clinically applicable at that time and maybe a bit of a stretch; we were focused at that time on how to use cytotoxic chemotherapy more effectively and safely. The "stretch" eventually became fulfilled prophecy, perfectly appropriate for the son of a rabbi.

Years later, I invited the now famous teacher and researcher to receive an award for his contributions to the field of neuro-oncology and oncology in general and to give a talk to our professional staff as well as to our interested patients and families. In preparation for introducing him, I read his biography "Dr. Folkman's War", R.Cooke, 2001, (which he autographed for me,) from cover to cover. He was impressed with my preparation, but I was inspired. Included in my comments were allusions to his stubborn persistence with a single idea which I said was typical more of surgeons than non-surgeons; it all comes down to Courage, not stubbornness. This "C" word, so lacking in so many ways these days, has come up multiple times in this tome. I also told the true story that he had saved all of his many grant rejections or "pink slips" and had them on display in the fellows' room so they could see what is required for success and not be deterred by the inevitable setbacks. Research is not the forte of many surgeons, but I do think the element of measured bravado and self-confidence seen in good surgeons is a valuable commodity for success in a very competitive field.

Judah humbly and eloquently presented his story of years of work with the same goal in mind, to elucidate the mechanism(s) by which tumors, and non-tumors, create new blood vessels, "neo-angiogenesis," to support their own growth. Until he began to get answers, he was much maligned by many for this work, but prevailed in the end. He worked out that the production of vascular endothelial growth factor (VEGF) under conditions of normal wound healing and abnormal tumor growth was the key. If that process could be blocked, tumors might literally be choked to death by inadequate blood supply. In theory, he was correct, and the drug bevacizumab was produced and eventually indicated for at least 7 types of cancer. Other targeted molecular therapies, mostly tyrosine kinase inhibitors, also included some effect on VEGF inhibition. Unfortunately, it wasn't as simple as he might have hoped. Most cancers were able to quickly evolve mechanisms to grow successfully despite the effective blockade of VEGF by bevacizumab. In the case of brain tumors, my area of interest, we called this type of growth co-optive as the tumors (not all) seemed to parasitize the existing normal microcirculation and continued to grow albeit more slowly and less destructively.

If Judah had not died unexpectedly at the height of his success, who knows where we might be now? For example, one of our speakers was a researcher from Genentech which produces bevacizumab (bev). When I asked what had been learned about mechanisms of tumor resistance to the drug, she *had no answer. We still don't. That question, I am certain, would be in the hands of Judah's best and brightest and would not have gone to dust with him. The shame of it all is that the immediate effect of bev on recurrent brain tumors is very dramatic and therapeutic. In some cases, it never wears off and long -term survival is the result, but most cases develop resistance, and we have no remedy for that. Ironically, the ability of tumors to evolve resistance to treatment is suicidal since the cancer dies with its host. I'm certain that this fact was not lost on Judah, and I can only imagine what Talmudic explanation he might have given.*

A few more words about bev before I close this chapter. The history of its use in brain tumors is of some interest. Many are of the opinion, which I believe to be incorrect, that bev does nothing more for brain tumor patients than reduce swelling and make a pretty picture of decreased contrast enhancement in MRIs, but fails to have any direct effect on the tumor itself. On the other hand, the other tumors for which bev is indicated do not have a problem of swelling or bright contrast on MRI imaging, so there must be something else going on. As I mentioned, I have cared for a sizable number of patients with glioblastoma, the median survival of which with standard therapy is 14.2 months, who have lived many years after recurrence under the influence of bev as their only therapy. Some appear to be cured and are off therapy. Again, things are never simple. Patients and tumors are heterogeneous.

A big problem with understanding the optimum use of bev is that, in most clinical trials, patients with large unresectable tumors have been excluded. In my experience, these are a subgroup most likely to benefit from this agent which often achieves rapid decrease in the volume of tumor and eliminates corticosteroid dependence which can be just as life-threatening as the tumor. In many cases, this benefit allows the patient to have other treatment sufficient to lengthen survival. A second subgroup of patients are those with gliomatosis cerebri who harbor widespread and multi-focal lower grade glioma which inevitably evolves focally to GBM. Use of bev in these patients seems to prevent this from happening or at least make it less likely. Again, no clinical trials have looked at this.

Finally, I would like to comment with some passion on two clinical trials which were done more or less concurrently to address the question of whether the addition of bev to standard chemotherapy with temozolomide would improve outcomes for patients with newly diagnosed glioblastoma. First, it must be understood that a test can be done on GBM tumor cells to determine if the gene for MGMT, a protein that reduces the efficacy of temozolomide (TMZ), is expressed or suppressed. To be fair, this is not a yes or no question, but clinical correlation is so strong between the result of this test and the response to TMZ that clinical trials must deal with this issue in order to produce meaningful results. In the two studies, patients were randomly assigned to get a standard course of TMZ with or without bev. Those that did not randomize to bev received a placebo infusion the ethics of which, just to be able to say that there was a placebo group, are questionable.

If one takes into consideration the fact that approximately 65% of patients can be predicted to get little or no benefit from TMZ, the study is confounding since only about 16% of patients would have received both an effective chemotherapy drug and bev. Nevertheless, the published conclusion was that bev adds nothing to TMZ for new patients. This conclusion nearly resulted in bev being disapproved for GBM altogether, but it was saved largely by the protests of Dr. Henry Friedman from Duke University who commands extraordinary respect. This is a classic example of a research standard being set that was unrealistic and became more important than the goal of finding better treatments for unfortunate patients. One if these studies was based at

MD Anderson Cancer Center and designed by their neuro-oncology group; they should know better. I want to be clear—the conclusions of the study are wrong, harmful to people, and nihilistic.

And so, the legacy of Judah Folkman continues. It is my contention that if he had survived long enough, he would have deserved and gotten the Nobel Prize for Medicine. Not bad for a rabbi's son from Cleveland, Ohio and a surgeon to boot.

Zichranah libracha (Hebrew for "rest in peace"). Courage is what it takes and what he had.

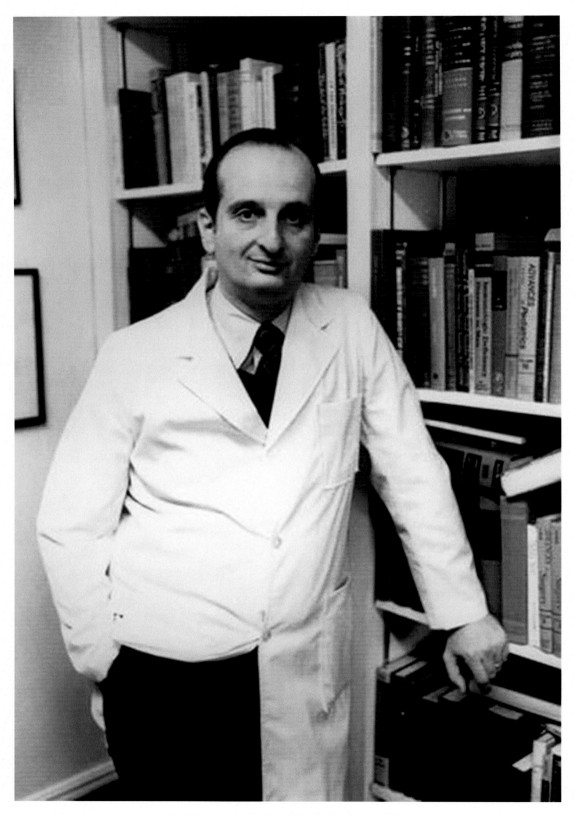

JUDAH FOLKMAN MD
With permission of Boston Children's Hospital

CHAPTER 15

Neurosurgeons I Have Known: Comedians, Cowards, Fools, Scoundrels, and *Mensches*

The following is a list of the neurosurgeons that I have worked with in my career in no particular order:

John Waldman, Larry Mc Cleary, Ken Winston, Michael Hitchcock, John McVicker, Timothy Fullagar, Karl Stecher, Paul Elliott, Jeffrey Masciopinto, Gary Van der Ark, Mark Robinson, J.D. Day, David Miller, Kevin Lillehei, Alex West, Dennis Volmer, Stewart Levy, Eric Parker, Adam Hebb, Marcus Keep, Raymond Sawaya, Mitchell Berger, Kris Smith, John Hudson, John Nichols, Michael Handler, Lloyd Mobley, Michael Rauzzino, Roderick Lamond, J. Adair Prall, Stephen Shogun, Alan Villavicenzio, Alan Waziri, Jeff Wisoff, Fred Epstein, Lee Krauth, Robert Spetzler, Paul Muller, Edward Oldfield, Shawn Markey, Steve Johnson, David Van Sickle, Linda Liang, Peter Syre

Of this extensive list of 44 neurosurgeons, let me make a few selective remarks. The first is that many of my medical colleagues would look at this list, at both its length as well as some of the surgeons, and ask how I had managed to avoid suicide. The following are those for whom I have the greatest respect and who have had the greatest impact:

Larry McCleary, *Mensch* 15- a very nice guy and a very good pediatric neurosurgeon. He was ambushed by another member of the list who publicly attacked him for doing what he believed to be necessary operations on children to correct early fusion of skull bones. This led to a deluge of lawsuits which probably had something to do with Larry having a massive heart attack which ended his career. Larry always called me to the operating room to see the anatomy of the tumors he operated on and to teach me neuro-anatomy in real time. He was much beloved by his patients and colleagues, your author included. The early end to his career, regardless of putative misdeeds, is a tragedy that deprived countless children of his love and skills.

Michael Hitchcock-a true *mensch* and gentleman who, with me, co-founded the CNI Center for Brain and Spinal Tumors shortly before his well -deserved retirement.

John McVicker-a fine neurosurgeon and a Scot who had some wild days in his familial homeland before settling into his career. We worked well together until he was badly treated by Swedish Hospital (join the club) and migrated to Colorado Springs. He specialized in deep brain stimulation for severe Parkinsonism, but was also an aggressive and skillful brain tumor surgeon. When he left, I gave him a painting of the Battle of Culloden as we drank a wee dram of Scotch. Inexplicably, we have never spoken since.

Timothy Fullagar- a real character and very good neurosurgeon now practicing in his wife's home state of Tennessee (guess who is the boss). One of the original crew in our Program at CNI, he spoke in a monotone, if at all, and realized that our Patient Care Coordinator and I were better choices than he to talk to his patients. His politics were just to the left of Louis XIV, but he was honest about it. He told me that he voted for the Colorado lottery because he knew that the money collected, mostly from the desperately poor, would help keep his mansion in open space.

J.D. Day-a brilliant and aggressive neurosurgeon renowned for asking several times at our brain tumor conference why the patient being discussed was not already in the operating room. He left Denver to became Chief of Neurosurgery at the University of Arkansas.

David Miller-nice guy and capable surgeon who was too tame for his dysfunctional practice and wisely left quickly for the mountains, but had already established himself for his dry sense of humor and wisdom which sounded like "Carlton the Doorman" from the television sitcom Rhoda.

Kevin Lillehei, Chief of Neurosurgery at University of Colorado and a superb neurosurgeon to whom I would have referred more patients, but didn't because I knew that his loyalty to his hospital was so great that he would steal the patients, and I would never see them again. Recently, however, he actually begged me to take a patient back that I had referred even though he knew I was retiring, because he had finally figured out that his neuro-oncologists would not provide aggressive care.

Alex West-a cranky, but talented neurosurgeon who was honest enough to admit to me that he would not do more aggressive or risky tumor removals at Swedish Hospital because the institution was not well respected enough to protect his reputation if something went wrong. No other neurosurgeon has ever admitted this to me.

A. Stewart Levy, *Mensch* 16, a CU-trained superb neurosurgeon and human being who, along with several members of his group, chose to refer patients with brain tumors to me even though I was at a competing hospital, because he believed I would provide the best care. This, I'm sure, cost him some political points, but the patients benefitted and so did I. I helped establish a brain tumor team at his hospital and faithfully attended brain tumor conference twice monthly for several years. Ultimately, he, like me, (what a coincidence,) was poorly treated by his hospital and joined Kaiser-Permanente where he was forced to give up many of our mutual patients much to my regret.

Marcus Keep-a very pleasant Canadian neurosurgeon with excellent credentials who often used the adjective, feral, to describe me since I was a bit off the beaten path. We enjoyed a very pleasant relationship for the short time he stayed until chased away by Dr. Elliott.

Raymond Sawaya-senior neurosurgeon at MD Anderson Cancer Center whom I invited to give one of our annual talks. He is a gentleman among men and was nice enough to put into words that ours was the best brain tumor program he had seen (other than his own of course).

Mitchell Berger, *Mensch* 13-Chief of Neurosurgery at University of California San Francisco to whom an entire chapter of this book is aptly devoted.

Kris Smith-a young and talented neurosurgeon from the Barrow Institute in Phoenix, Arizona whom I met at the annual meeting of the Rocky Mountain Neurosurgical Society. He specializes in laser-guided neurosurgery and use of the ketogenic diet in brain cancer treatment.

John Hudson-a partner of Stewart Levy who has shared numerous patients with me and has provided excellent care. He is the only one of his group that is still at St. Anthony's Hospital in Lakewood, Colorado and has agreed to accept patients to follow once I retire.

John Nichols-also partners with Drs. Levy and Hudson who demonstrated exceptional compassion in his neurosurgical practice and actively sought the advice of his respected colleagues.

Alan Waziri, a Columbia U. -trained bright young neurosurgeon of Afghani ancestry on the CU faculty who defied his superiors by referring several patients to me instead of his own neuro-oncologists because he believed my superior outcome data. He fell into disfavor and moved back east.

Jeffrey Wisoff-a senior neurosurgeon at NYU who trained other neurosurgeons with whom I have worked including Ben Rubin. He was a colleague of mine on the Brain Tumor Strategy Group of the Children's Cancer Group who told the unforgettable story of an insane patient who jumped out of the window of Belleview Hospital in New York and landed on the hood of his car, whereupon Jeff got out and treated him in the alley. He spearheaded a study which helped clarify the outcomes and best treatment approaches for children with low grade gliomas.

Fred Epstein-a well-known and flamboyant NYU neurosurgeon who was famous for his ability to do very risky operations on the brainstem and spinal cord who, unfortunately, died in a bicycle accident in New York. I knew him well enough to refer a young boy with a brainstem tumor with the expectation that he would tell the family that no operation could be done. Tragically, he did an operation which left the boy neurologically devastated for the rest of his life. He couldn't say no because he cared and overestimated his skills, but knew better.

Paul Muller-a Canadian neurosurgeon with whom we did an interesting study using photodynamic therapy in malignant brain tumor patients. He was one of our lecturers. Unfortunately, poor study design prevented the success of an exciting study on which we collaborated using a light-sensitive chemical to improve local control of brain tumors.

Edward Oldfield-a well- respected neurosurgeon at the NIH, another of our lecturers, who pioneered a system to gently infuse treatment for brain tumors directly into the brain, a system which might eventually bear fruit.

Benjamin Rubin, *Mensch* 17-a young, personable, and very skillful neurosurgeon, trained by Dr. Wisoff at NYU, who had the Courage to refer patients to me instead of the neuro-oncologist that had been recruited by Swedish Hospital, without my knowledge or input, to replace me (even though I had no plans to retire). He has been a joy to work with and has just made a decision to migrate to another hospital leaving me and my patients behind for a very good reason, I'm sure.

The fact that many of these noteworthy neurosurgeons qualify in my book as *mensches,* given my high standards for this title, is quite remarkable. That is why I didn't take my own life, or at least one reason. Among the others for whom I have less enthusiasm were three who didn't do operations that needed to be done, two who did operations that shouldn't have been done, one who did inadequate operations that he called adequate, one who left his post to go find a rare bird and lost his privileges, one who operated on one of my patients and refused to tell the patient that she had a stroke, and a few who were just prototypically unpleasant.

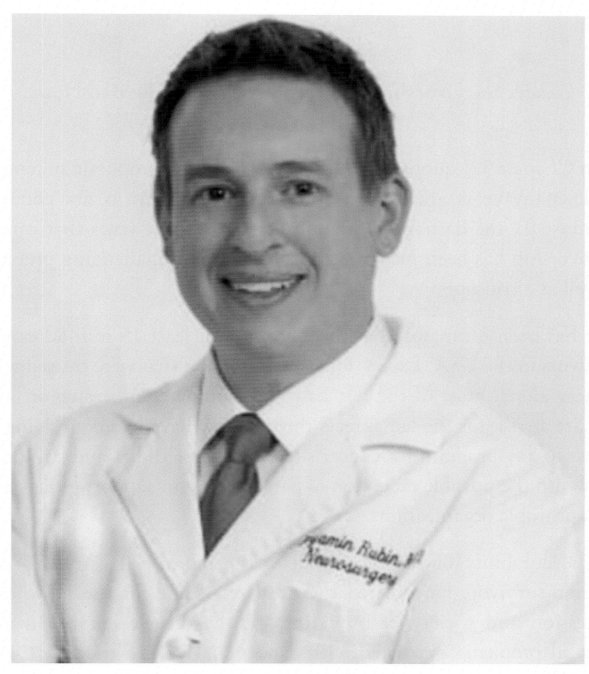

BENJAMIN RUBIN MD
Photo with permission of Dr. Rubin

CHAPTER 16

Cancer Survivorship, the Good News and the Bad News

In Chapter 5, I quoted Dr. Giulio D'Angio in a prophetic statement made many years ahead of its time. He said "Cure is not enough; we must fix the damage". It is only in the last few years that cancer survivorship has been recognized, ironically, as a challenging problem as well as a triumph.

It has been estimated that there are now at least 15 million cancer survivors in the USA. Except for a small fraction that were treated with surgery alone, most of the rest had radiation, chemotherapy, or both and are at risk for the late effects thereof. Few have had counseling or access to any program for cancer survivors; these didn't and still don't exist with the possible exception of participation in support groups and philanthropic organizations.

The curability of cancer as well as the increase in survival time for non-survivors has created the great challenge for the healthcare profession and society of providing for the diverse emotional and physical problems associated with cancer survival. In the late 1970s, Gerald Koocher, a PhD psychologist, wrote a book about childhood leukemia survivors called "The Damocles Syndrome: Psychosocial Consequences of Surviving Childhood Cancer," which described the heavy emotional burden carried by childhood leukemia survivors, a complex burden which includes the guilt which is unavoidable when a patient survives, but knows others that do not. This is very similar to the guilt experienced by military combat survivors, and the syndrome of PTSD, with which they are too often afflicted, and variably occurs in the childhood cancer survivors as well. Whereas society has at least made an attempt, with limited success, to lighten the burden on the soldiers, almost nothing has been done for their similarly burdened childhood and adult comrades who are cancer survivors.

Just a few years ago, about 2013, Dan Miller, who was at that time the Chief Operating Officer at Swedish Medical Center, offered me the position of Director of Cancer Survivors' Services. He did this in part because the hospital's cancer program was mandated to create such a program and in part because he realized that I had been mistreated by the hospital and wished to make amends for the damage that had been done to my livelihood (and ego of course). I think he also believed that I was the most qualified MD available to do this because of my long and diverse career as a cancer doctor.

I, like most of my colleagues, had recognized the need for such a program, but had little knowledge or resources with which to take action and no opportunity. I was given the opportunity and tried to make the best of it. I read virtually everything I could find on the subject which was quite limited. I also reviewed the guidelines which had been created by the NCCN which mostly focused on tumor surveillance rather than the scars of cancer survival. I reviewed hundreds of charts to get a sense of what, if anything, was already being done and found almost nothing. I had meetings with patients to get a sense of their experience. Very few showed up, but those that did taught me that they were largely unaware of the effects of their survivorship or were overtly suffering with no idea what to do about it. I found most of the doctors who cared for these patients to be either uninterested or too busy to be helpful. I hatched the idea of setting up a clinic focused on cancer survivors which would provide comprehensive care for these patients, both emotional and physical, to identify and mitigate the late effects of treatment as well as attending to the very real issue of avoidance or early detection of other cancers.

Unfortunately, my position was dissolved without warning, explanation, apology, or any indication of appreciation of my efforts. By that time, Dan Miller was gone, deservedly promoted and moved to another facility.

Quite coincidentally, I was offered at that time an opportunity to become involved in the shiny new hyperbaric oxygen program at the hospital, a joint venture between Swedish Medical Center and a private company called NexGen Hyperbaric founded by its visionary CEO, Jonathan Rotella. I believe that Dan Miller also had a hand in this just before being promoted and departing for another hospital. This opportunity, whether accidental or visionary, turned out to be of great importance for me personally and for many cancer survivors. Let me provide a brief primer about hyperbaric oxygen therapy (HBOT).

It has been known for more than a hundred years that, if oxygen is breathed under more than atmospheric pressure, very high levels of oxygen will dissolve in the blood as it passes through the lungs. Initially this was used to keep patients alive during cardiac surgery, but this use was replaced by cardiopulmonary bypass. Later, HBOT was used to treat the bends caused by diving mishaps in which nitrogen bubbles form during ascent and cause terrible pain and tissue injury. Other emergency uses included air or gas embolism, cyanide poisoning, and carbon monoxide poisoning. More recently, with the development of single person chambers (monoplace) as opposed to multiple person chambers (multiplace), it has become feasible to treat patients with more chronic problems such as diabetic wounds and radiation injury. Patients can receive 100% oxygen safely and comfortably in these chambers, and can be treated for many weeks as outpatients.

What non-healing wounds and radiation damage have in common is injury to and depletion of small blood vessels which we call microcirculation. Such tissues are deprived of oxygen (hypoxia) as well as nutrition. In the case of wounds, this impairs healing, and in the case of radiation, the injured tissues are unhealthy which can produce pain, bleeding, poor healing of surgical wounds, and, in the case of the brain, a variety of deficits depending on the part of the brain that was radiated. The repair of damaged microcirculation by HBOT is caused by an artificially enlarged oxygen gradient between healthy and unhealthy tissue which stimulates production of factors, especially vascular endothelial growth factor (VEGF, see tribute to Judah Folkman), which induces the production of new microcirculation (neo-angiogenesis). This improves the oxygenation and nutrition of these tissues and promotes restoration of normal function and improvement in most of the symptoms detailed above. The degree of benefit depends greatly on the viability of the damaged tissue, something that many do not fully understand, i.e. dead is dead.

Once I was trained and began supervising patients who were receiving HBOT, including several that were being treated for radiation injury, I realized that this treatment might benefit a large number, perhaps a hundred or more, of my brain tumor survivors who had been treated with radiation therapy and were experiencing neurological deterioration.

I looked into the literature and found almost nothing. A pivotal paper published by J. Niezgoda et al in 2016 that summarized the results of several thousand cancer patients treated with HBOT indicated that only about 2% of all treated patients had brain tumors. Thus, very little was known about the use of HBOT in brain tumor patients. Fortunately, the indication for HBOT for radiation soft tissue injury was not specific for any tissue and thus my brain tumor patients were eligible.

We started out with a very conservative approach to ensure that brain tumor patients could tolerate HBOT, and our expectations were low. We hoped to slow or stop the progressive deterioration of brain function that had been observed, but had no inkling that some patients might actually improve or that the improvement would be sustained. We also started with the most severely affected patients many of whom had received radiation many years before their HBOT. Our initial approach used lower than optimum pressure and limited numbers of treatments. We were particularly concerned about oxygen-induced seizures. As it turned out, we did not see any evidence of increased risk of seizures or any other unexpected side effects. Once we knew this, we increased the pressure to 2.4 times sea level (ATA), equivalent to about 40 feet of sea water, and began extending the number of treatments from 30 to 60 or more. Once we did this, we were stunned by the results.

Instead of merely slowing the patients' decline, we actually saw very significant functional improvement of many different symptoms. The clinical improvement correlated virtually 100% with easily recognized improvement by MRI imaging which showed evidence of vascular repletion, some examples of which are shown here: (the level of blood volume in the brain correlates with the color; green is better than blue).

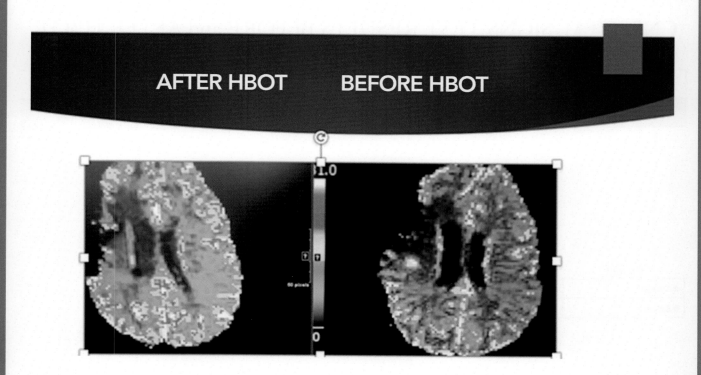

AFTER HBOT   BEFORE HBOT

EVIDENCE OF VASCULAR REPLETION DEMONSTRATED BY COLOR PERFUSION MRI IMAGING

Patients were tested by neuropsychologists before HBOT to quantify and characterize their deficits. It was our intention to repeat this testing after HBOT, but the testing was expensive and arduous, so many patients were not re-tested. When they were, the results were difficult to correlate with clinical and imaging improvement. Recently, we have acquired software called CNS Vital Signs which allows online cognitive testing which is inexpensive, takes only about 40 minutes, and provides immediate reports which are elegant and quantitative. Thus far, we have seen several patients whose repeat testing on CNS Vital Signs demonstrated meaningful improvement which correlated well with our clinical observations. This type of testing in no way replaces or is an adequate substitute for formal testing by a qualified neuro-psychologist, but lends itself well to serial testing.

CNS VITAL SIGNS TEST RESULTS BEFORE and AFTER HBOT

CNS Vital Signs Graphical Report

Above Average	Average	Low Average	Low	Very Low

Patient	Test Time	Neurocognitive Index	Composite Memory	Verbal Memory	Visual Memory	Psychomotor Speed	Reaction Time	Complex Attention	Cognitive Flexibility	Processing Speed	Executive Function	Simple Attention	Motor Speed
◆	Before HBOT	53	55	48	79	63	31	65	50	75	52	107	70
◆	After HBOT	74	61	80	89	87	63	65	76	78	85	107	97

We have presented our data from these brain tumor patients at several national and international meetings and are preparing a manuscript for publication. We have learned that: HBOT at 2.4 ATA for 90 minutes is safe in radiated brain tumor patients; 60 treatments are required to produce sustainable benefit; treatment more than 100 months after radiation is less likely to be beneficial; improvement in a wide variety of symptoms related to brain injury was observed clinically and verified by both cognitive testing and color perfusion imaging on MRI scans.

Despite claims by a number of hyperbaric oxygen providers that durable benefit is seen in patients with a variety of chronic brain injury conditions including traumatic brain injury (TBI), I am on record and firm in my conclusion that radiation injury is the only chronic and progressive brain condition for which there are compelling data which indicate that there is treatment, HBOT, which produces sustained improvement rather than temporary slowing of the disease. I would predict, however, that patients with vascular dementia, of which there are many times more than patients with radiation injury to brain, as well as selected patients with TBI if properly treated, would benefit equally, but there are insufficient data yet to prove this.

And so there you have it, the events which led to my interest in cancer survivorship, "fixing the damage", and the good fortune of finding myself in a new field, hyperbaric oxygen medicine, which turned out to be unexpectedly and dramatically beneficial to my own brain tumor survivors and, hopefully, many more around the world. Of all my accomplishments in a long career, this is probably the most meaningful and most likely to be my legacy. Sometimes it just comes down to being in the right place at the right time and having the sense to know it. "Being useful" is not always accomplished by intent alone, but often requires an opportunity which I certainly had and for which I am ever grateful. I thank Dan Miller and Jonathan Rotella for intentionally or intuitively giving me the opportunity. Despite my forthcoming criticism of corporate medicine, these men are examples of how different it could be if the corporate "suits", most of whom are not medically trained, understand that people's lives depend on their decisions.

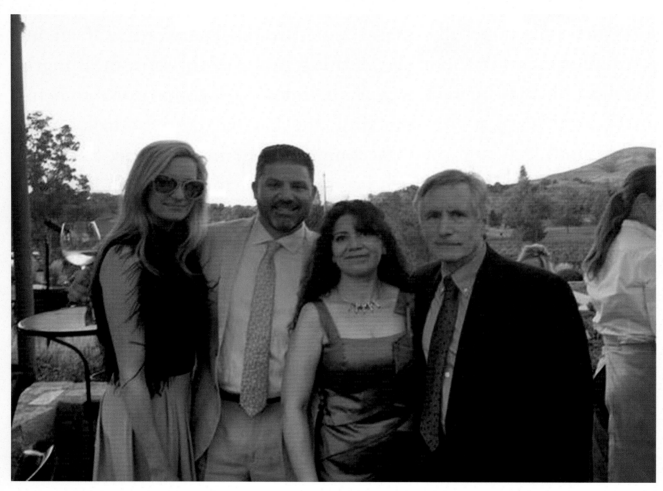

THE ROTELLAS (LEFT)AND THE ARENSONS (RIGHT)

CHAPTER 17

In Which I Hold Forth on the Ups and Downs of What You Have Just Read

In these chapters, I have recounted the details of my own nearly five decades as a cancer doctor as well as the many important events that occurred during that time. Some of these were personal and some more universal in their impact. It has been a varied and rich career which is sadly in its autumn (or early winter). With this experience in hand, I would like to take the liberty to hold forth briefly on the changes, both good and bad, which I have observed. I'm certain that my view would not be shared by all of my medical colleagues, but I think I have earned this opportunity to speak out.

From a scientific point of view, the progress which has taken place since I finished medical school is next to miraculous. At that time, Watson and Crick and just worked out the structure of DNA. Now we have mapped the entire human genome and developed the means of identifying and targeting the genes involved in cancer. We have brought the cure rate of childhood cancer, mostly through the use of combination cytotoxic chemotherapy, to 85%. We have also dramatically enlarged the arsenal of treatments available for cancer and improved survival and quality of survival. We have developed a greater knowledge of the role of the immune system in cancer treatment although it is more limited than we had hoped. We have had enough success to have created a massive need for a better program for more than 15 million cancer survivors.

So, what do I have to complain about? First, let me review some of the reasons why we have made such tremendous progress in cancer knowledge and treatment, and then move on to some reasons why we haven't done better.

I focused a good deal of this saga on the cure of childhood leukemia and other pediatric tumors. This achievement was made by a relatively small cadre of medical professionals who understood their daunting task and were willing to do what needed to be done. They were willing to accept failure, watch patients die from their therapy rather than their disease, take calculated risks, and exercise flexibility and creativity on a daily basis to cope with the heterogeneity of the patients and their diseases. The most crucial human quality necessary to do these things was and is Courage. As well, creativity and flexibility are crucial qualities as was the case when the National Wilms Tumor Study was formed and when it was decided to combine vincristine and actinomycin D instead of single agent treatment for Wilms tumor.

Now let me expound upon the current situation. While the technology and scientific knowledge base has increased exponentially, the patient outcomes have not. The most common adult cancers, prostate, breast, lung, and colorectal are still incurable once they have spread, and together these cancers result in close to a million deaths per year in this country alone. Survival has been extended, at enormous expense, but cure remains elusive

In the context of these unpleasant facts, the cost of care for these patients has skyrocketed. Targeted molecular therapies, which are palliative in all but rare cases, and immunotherapy, also palliative, are enormously expensive and have a panoply of side effects which are more difficult to manage in many cases than the side effects of conventional chemotherapy. These newer agents are so expensive that they have essentially ended the era of private practices of oncology. Instead, oncologists, both pediatric and adult, are employed either by hospitals or corporations such as U.S. Oncology or Kaiser-Permanente where their practice of oncology is controlled by their employers and creativity and risk-taking is stifled.

While it is true that, for a short time, private practices of medical oncology were very profitable, that era ended quickly when the prices of drugs went up and reimbursement went down, more or less simultaneously. The reason why these practices were so profitable before this perfect storm of calamities occurred is that they were infinitely more efficient and economical than inpatient therapy which had been the standard. In addition, and very importantly, these practices provided an environment where oncologists had the freedom to treat their patients as individuals and to be creative in the use of available therapies.

In this environment, medical decisions were evidence-based and sometimes more intuitive and experiential. For example, it is known that vinca alkyloids such as vincristine, vinblastine, and vinorelbine are anti-mitotic drugs that cross the blood/brain barrier and have activity against most brain tumors. In recurrent glioblastoma, I frequently used vinorelbine for palliation in the absence of better options even if there were few, if any, studies to support this treatment. Several patients responded well enough to live for more than a year whereas their predicted survival was perhaps 2-4 months. There was not sufficient interest, (generic drug and therefore little profit,) or patients to do a phase II study with vinorelbine, but there is no doubt in my mind that this is a useful drug and worth a try in selected patients. Now, even in the very few private practices that survive, the use of this drug would be impossible.

Another anecdote that highlights this line of thinking is the first use of bevacizumab (bev) for recurrent glioblastoma (GBM). Dr Virginia Stark Vance, who has a private practice of neuro-oncology in Texas, decided that it might help one of her recurrent GBM patients to give bev since it had shown activity in other malignancies through its anti-angiogenesis effect, especially since GBM is known to demonstrate vascular proliferation as well as production of high levels of VEGF which bev inhibits. She was able to use the drug because Dr. Henry Friedman at Duke had enough clout and some early data to get her the drug. To make a long story short, the response was rapid and dramatic, and bev was eventually approved for use in recurrent GBM. In this context why is it so rare now to observe the phenomenon I just described?

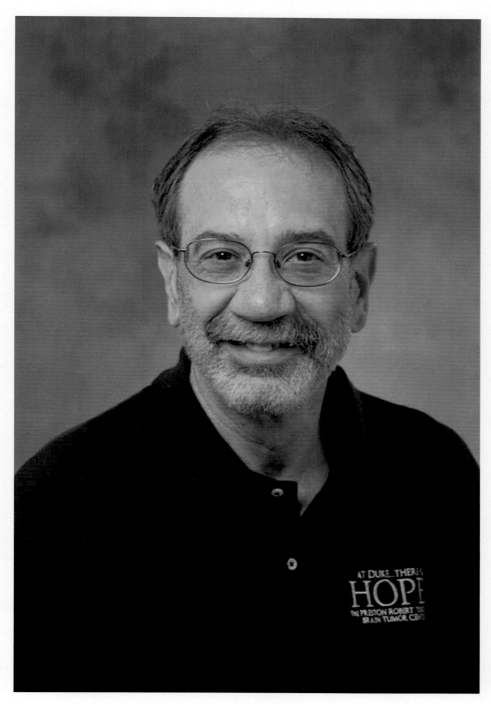

DR. HENRY FRIEDMAN, *Mensch* 18
Obtained from Dr. Friedman with permission to publish

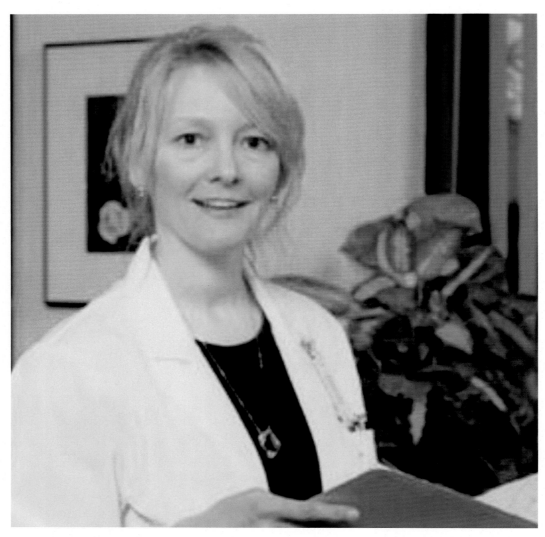

VIRGINIA STARK VANCE MD
Photo provided by Dr. Vance with permission to publish

As mentioned above, private practices, in which oncologists had the most flexibility to practice the "art" of individualizing treatment, have been essentially eliminated by the cash flow issues created by the cost of newer therapies as well as reduced reimbursement. These practices have very high overhead associated with the requirement for many skilled professionals and space in which to do infusions. It has simply become untenable to keep them going. Instead, most oncologists are now employees of hospitals and corporations both of which have a clear bottom line of profitability. They will not allow oncologists to be "artists" for fear of non-reimbursement or jeopardizing their reputation. I was told recently by a colleague from New York City that there was not a single private practice of medical oncology left in greater New York.

Now that I have told the facts of the current state of oncology, I will ask the rhetorical question of whether we are better off than we were a decade or two ago. The answer is unclear. Patients are living longer, although not necessarily better, but cure remains very rare in the most common malignancies of adults, The reason for this is multi-factorial, but I would assert that the combination of greed on the part of those that make the drugs and pay the doctors, and lack of Courage on the part of the doctors themselves, as well as lack of creativity, has degraded the progress that we all anticipated.

I don't mean to suggest that medicine is the only area of society where the combination of greed and cowardice has stifled progress. Take a look at the current political climate, the climate itself, the state of the world economically and politically, religious corruption, business, including IT and social media which produce obscene profits while, with a few notable exceptions, return little to society. These all have the same common denominators, (forgive me one more time,) greed and cowardice. It is, however, most painful to me to see the influence of these negatives on the medical profession since it has been my life's passion and remains so.

Just a few words to clarify what I mean by Courage, or cowardice, the lack thereof. What I don't mean is the kind of courage we associate with military heroes, firemen, etc. i.e. the willingness to risk one's life for some higher cause. What I do mean is the willingness to take the relatively small risk of making less money or being subjected to criticism in order to improve the outcome of patients. In some cases, as I discussed in more detail in my chapter on neurosurgeons, it is simply the willingness to do what is universally considered appropriate, but carries the risk of an occasional bad outcome. It also means having the confidence, based on evidence and experience, to treat patients creatively as individuals and not simply follow "guidelines". Of course, this might involve some extra time and work, but that is what doctors do, or should do. At least that is what I was taught, and I have never been criticized by anyone for hard work on behalf of my patients even though it certainly contributed to my two failed marriages and adversely affected my children.

I can't conclude this diatribe without reference to humor. I have given some examples of humor in this book without which my colleagues and I would never have survived as long as we did in our very challenging field of medicine. Those that are both courageous and creative invariably find humor in their work, no matter how taxing it might be. Shakespeare prototypically used humor to offset some of his tragic plots. The presence of a sense of humor, in my experience, indicates humility which is a necessary component of Courage. The lack of humor is always worrisome; take a look at politics as an example: how many times have Richard Nixon or Donald Trump made you laugh?

Because I have witnessed and reported many events in my own career in which great things were accomplished by those who had the Courage to put the cure of cancer and reduction of suffering ahead of personal gain, I have not lost hope and, just as in those early days when I was informed as a cancer doctor, I know things will get better, because they simply can't get much worse. As Igor (actor Marty Feldman) famously stated in Mel Brooks' classic movie, Young Frankenstein, "It could be worse, it could be raining." after which, of course, they were caught in a deluge, but things finally worked out after a brain transplant.

CHAPTER 18

The Story of Mark, Claire, and Caryn in Which Tragedy Begets Love

About 7 years ago, a new patient with a partially removed glioblastoma named Claire Alpert was referred to me. She was a charming blond, an accomplished musician who played piano and organ for her church although she had converted to Judaism in Baltimore's leading conservative congregation. She was in her 50s, fully functional, and based on those facts and the successful tumor surgery, was predicted to have a relatively good prognosis. She sailed through her early treatment with radiation and two chemotherapy drugs, but once on monthly post-radiation treatment, developed persistent low blood counts which radically limited her treatment and jeopardized her predicted longer survival.

I had recently joined a conservative Jewish synagogue, Hebrew Educational Alliance (HEA), which was more traditional than my previous affiliations, but my fiancée, now wife Aura, preferred a more traditional congregation. She had converted to Judaism for her first marriage in an orthodox program, and her beloved first mother-in-law of blessed memory, Helen Beckenstein Pilcer, had kept a strict Jewish home. Aura had been Helen's favorite, and Aura had devoted herself to Helen during her losing battle with early onset Alzheimer's disease. Helen was a hero of the holocaust, a member of the famous Beilski

Partisans who had escaped death at Auschwitz to help with the Russian resistance against the Nazis, and spoke seven languages.

I was standing in a line near the altar because we had a tradition of stepping forward to name anyone for whom we wanted to pray for healing at a certain part of the ceremony. I noticed a tall, handsome man in front of me in line whom I hadn't met. When his turn came, he named "Claire Alpert, my wife". "Coincidentally", I was also there to ask for Claire's healing. That is how I met Claire's husband Mark with whom I am still good friends. He would come with Claire for appointments and ask very intelligent questions; he was an engineer. He often brought me a copy of the Forward to which he subscribed. The Forward is a relic newspaper published in New York founded to serve the immigrant Jewish population there, especially the Yiddish -speaking eastern Europeans.

As time went by, Claire's disease returned and progressed, and she ultimately succumbed. Mark was devastated, but managed; he has several adult children and grandchildren and didn't have the luxury of being paralyzed by his grief. Of course, he became an eligible bachelor very quickly, but wasn't ready. Sometime in 2016, however, he started seeing a divorced congregant of HEA by the name of Caryn Grossman. By the end of the year, it was clear that they were a couple, but also clear that any idea of marriage was premature, no doubt related to the children of each who needed more time to be won over. We invited Mark and Caryn to spend New Year's Eve with us and chose to see a concert at the Denver Performing Arts Center followed by a late dinner at Hotel Monaco's Café Panzano in Denver. This is where Aura and I became engaged, also on New Year's Eve, in 2011. After a great dinner, we walked back to our downtown homes, one of which we used as guest quarters. Fireworks erupted; it was midnight and 2017.

Their relationship continued, and Caryn proved herself up to the formidable task of being accepted by Mark's children. Mark did the same. Caryn was stalwart in her empathy for his loss which he talked about often. To make a long story short, it worked. Mark had found love out of his grief. In this case, his new love was a woman who could share his love for his Jewish heritage even though his children were less enthusiastic.

Just a few months ago, Mark and Caryn got married under a *chuppah* in a traditional Jewish ceremony. It was, as you might expect, a very emotional event. I was there of course, in the front row of the sanctuary, completely overwhelmed with a combination of happiness and exultation in spite of the very palpable level of tension on the faces of the two families. For me, this was one of those life-affirming events that keep me going by proving that something positive can come from the worst of tragedies, that all the losses I have witnessed have had at least that possibility. The new Alperts honeymooned in the Canadian Maritimes, the place where Aura and I have purchased a property, (McNab's Cove, Cape Breton,) and plan to spend a good deal of our time once I am finally and fully "retired".

I suppose it is possible that all these unlikely nexuses could be purely coincidence, but I doubt it. For me, they are simply proof that there is something about our life on earth, with all its contradictions and unanswerable questions, that has meaning. Call it what you want, you won't be proven wrong.

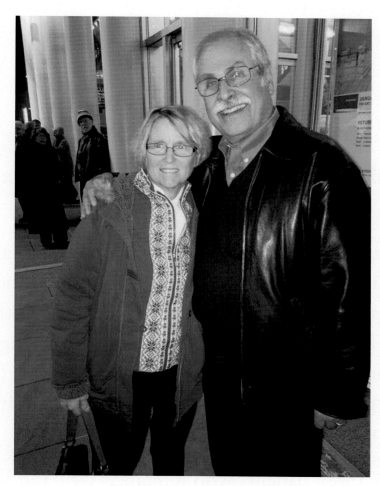

MARK AND CLAIRE

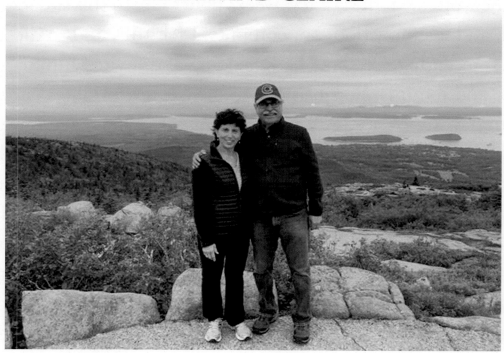

MARK AND CARYN HONEYMOONING

CHAPTER 19

The Story of Rita and Doug, Making the Best of a Bad Deal

I recently lost a patient with glioblastoma, Rita Buys, a beautiful and charismatic woman with a devoted and loving husband, Doug. The Buys were people of faith, but faith which included other faiths and philosophies. They were patently "in love" despite being in their early 60s. Rita will be one of the last of my beloved patients, (not all fit this description,) to pass away since I am on the verge of closing my practice of neuro-oncology.

Rita is one of those patients who remained well and herself in every sense of the word until the last few weeks of her life. In this situation, death is surreal, and it simply does not compute. I felt this, and so did Doug. I called him recently to see how he was doing and invited him to come by the office and reminisce or just be together. A few minutes later he was there. Our day was over, so Aura, (who is my office manager as well as my domestic boss,) and I were able to lock the door and sit down with Doug in privacy and quiet. He told us that he was struggling, but spending a great deal of time with his daughter which had been very helpful. His faith had sustained him. He hadn't changed anything since Rita's death. All her things were in place, and he was in no hurry to change that. As we reviewed these things, he said something that I had never heard before from a grieving spouse, even though I had often counseled patients to prioritize and intensify their lives in the face of a shortened prognosis.

Doug said that Rita's illness had been a gift in which the fatal diagnosis had led them to spend the last two years of their life together more meaningfully and intimately than ever before. This is the way it should be, but often isn't for understandable reasons.

Most patients fight their disease, even when they are told that they cannot be cured, to the end. In this fight, there is no time or energy left for anything that could be described as "intimacy". I have even tried to use math to make my point. I ask patients to give me a number between 1 and 10 to describe how much more meaningful life has become since their diagnosis. Most will give a high number once they think about it. If their realistic survival goal is two years, we multiply their number, 9 for example, times 2 and get 18. I tell the patient that, if lived to the fullest, they have the equivalent of 18 years to live. For many, this makes sense. However, it is easier said than done. In Doug and Rita's case, they actually did it. Doug thanked us profusely for providing him and Rita with the opportunity for this to happen. His gratitude is genuine, and so is mine for being given the opportunity.

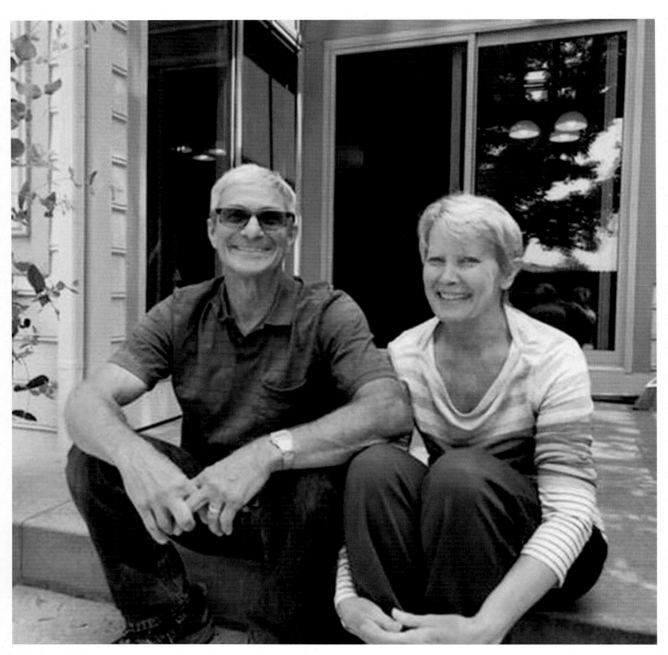

DOUG AND RITA BUYS

Chapter 20

"Urology, Please Hold"

It wasn't until I decided to have a vasectomy after the birth of my fourth child that I had much to do with urologists. I did cross path with a pediatric urologist or two during my time as a pediatric oncologist. One, whom I met at Albany Medical College, was an ambitious and strongly Catholic young Irishman who tragically attempted to remove an unresectable, (cannot be safely removed,) kidney tumor from a child. During the procedure, he inadvertently tied off an artery that supplied the liver with blood, and the child died of liver failure. He would probably have survived his kidney tumor which we could have shrunk with radiation and chemotherapy and made the surgery much safer. As far as I know, the tumor, along with the hepatic artery with a ligature around it, still resides in the pathology lab at Albany Medical Center as an unspoken warning.

A few years later, now living in Denver, Colorado, I saw an adult urologist to have a vasectomy. I arrived with high anxiety, but he was very efficient and managed to inject me with 10 milligrams of valium intravenously shortly after my arrival. I felt nothing and remembered nothing until he showed me what he had removed and asked if I was satisfied. I couldn't have been more satisfied and relieved, and after he turned away to do some charting, I left the treatment room and went to the front desk dressed in a jockstrap and a backless paper gown where I began signing patients in until one of the receptionists, laughing hysterically, coaxed me back into the treatment room. Needless to say, the next day, with swelling, pain, and no valium, was much less enjoyable.

Later, I began seeing the same urologist for an enlarging prostate and rising PSA, a test for blood levels of a protein which correlates with the size of the prostate and may be elevated in prostate cancer. I continued with him for several years and several prostate biopsies until one was finally positive for prostate cancer at the lowest detectable level of risk. He advised me to have this treated in his facility by a type of radiation called cyberknife which focuses the radiation precisely enough to allow only 5 instead of about 30 treatments with less focused radiation. I went to see the radiation oncologist, subsequently replaced, who recommended the therapy and assured me that the morbidity of the treatment would be low.

Because I had already been through this process with my father-in-law, I knew that careful surveillance, rather than therapy, was a safe option and that the morbidity of any form of radiation can be severe with involvement of bladder and rectum and impotence all possible. Because I was not given the option to do surveillance, and because the cyberiknife treatment is owned by the urologist and his group, I got a second opinion and am still under vigilant surveillance without treatment under the care of a different urologist. Since that time, I have treated numerous patients for radiation injury after prostate radiation, including cyberknife, using hyperbaric oxygen. This is an effective treatment described in more detail in another chapter, but usually there is some permanent damage. This brings up a subject worth discussing in more detail.

Although I have a urologist whom I trust and like, and there are many more like him, the field itself has a problem the solution of which is elusive. That is, they have a vested interest in being the exclusive providers of care for a very large population of men who either have or are at risk for prostate cancer. The entire process, from surveillance to biopsies, then possible diagnosis and, finally, treatment, is done by the urologists who are often superb surgeons, but certainly not oncologists. This situation is analogous to the one described elsewhere in this manuscript in which neurologists, both by intention and default, have taken over the field of neuro-oncology, the treatment of brain tumors, without training in oncology. In both cases, I believe this is an unhealthy situation.

Oncologists are trained in the complete management of cancer patients which includes diagnosis, treatment, palliation, end-of-life care—in other words, the complete management of the patient's physical, emotional, and even financial challenges. Oncologists invariably work as part of a team which is required to deal with such diverse issues effectively. On the other hand, urologists have not been versed in this model, nor have neurologists. Thus, their patients often get suboptimum care. Moreover, in the case of urologists, they often own and benefit financially from some form of radiation therapy which, understandably, they promote as superior to other approaches with little or no data to support their claim.

Furthermore, once they have purchased expensive equipment and hired a radiation oncologist to treat the patients, they are likely to treat patients who might not need to be treated, especially those, like me, who have minimal prostate tumor burden. Needless to say, the radiation therapy is very lucrative. This issue is a big controversy in the medical field in which one side overtreats to avoid the risk of missing an opportunity to cure the patient while the other side is very concerned about the consequences, both medical and financial, of overtreating men who could instead be followed carefully and many of whom would never need to be treated. The morbidity of treatment, both surgical and radiation, is more often than not underestimated, but once done, the patient must deal with it for the rest of his life.

My opinion is that urologists' involvement should be limited to diagnosis and surgery, while radiation and chemotherapy should be done by full- service oncologists who are likely to be more holistic in their approach and more concerned about the consequences of therapy. Oncologists usually do not benefit financially from radiation while radiation oncologists, who get most of their referrals from oncologists, do derive financial benefit, but have a broad source of referrals and treat many types of cancer. They are, therefore, more likely to be objective and more honest with prostate cancer patients than radiation oncologists who exclusively treat prostate cancer and are employed by urologists.

Aside from these "minor" concerns, I am very fond of urologists who clearly have the best jokes of all medical specialists and the expertise and ability to assist men in a variety of lucrative ways to maintain sexual function as long as possible (please excuse the pun).

Chapter 21

How My Jewishness Affected My Medical Career (and Life)

If you believe the genetic testing service, 23 and Me, I am genetically 100% Ashkenazi Jew. This was no surprise to me and a waste of money and time. Nevertheless, from an ancestral point of view, that is what I am. There are many others with the same ancestry whose lives are unaffected or minimally affected by it. That is not the case with me.

Jews that practice the Jewish religion, which is optional, have been exposed to a complex and ancient, some say sacred, set of principles, *(mitzvot,* commandments and *middot,* virtuous behaviors,) by which they are expected to live. These include 613 commandments, not just 10, all spelled out in the Five Books of Moses, the Torah, which provide a code to live by and which, if followed, guarantee a life well lived. There are 48 *middot.* Of course, many of the commandments have been altered to be appropriate for modernity, and some are no longer relevant; e.g. what justice must be done if your neighbor's ox falls into your well.

There is no question that this code has had a major impact on my behavior, especially in medicine. It all boils down to one *mitvah,* "that which is repugnant to you, do not do to others".

In the Christian world this is The Golden Rule. Jews, somewhat Chauvinistically, like to say that they spend their time learning how to live while Christians spend their time professing a faith in hopes of getting to Heaven, a place that no one knows exists. The key word is "know".

In the practice of medicine, it is crucial to "know" as much as possible in order to practice based on evidence and not faith. That is not to say that we can know everything, and therefore sometimes we must make decisions based on our best guess. This guess is more likely to be the correct one if we are as knowledgeable and experienced as possible. The word "know" is a bit tricky since, in medicine and many other things, new information can change things that we thought we "knew". Thus, humility, flexibility, and an open mind are crucial.

Having said that, the issue of fact vs faith comes up daily in my medical practice; this has been the case for many years. At first, I took a hard line when patients suggested remedies that lacked any scientific basis. I knew that they would resort to these "absurdities" regardless of my opinion, but at least I wouldn't be blamed for supporting them. Over time, and I suppose with greater maturity, I began to take a less critical approach in which I explained the relative risks vs the unlikely benefits. I often used the example of B vitamins which actually accelerated the progression of childhood leukemia. This ultimately led to the development of an effective chemotherapy drug, methotrexate, which worked by interfering with the stimulation of leukemic cells by the B vitamin folic acid.

Magical thinking, or faith-based decision making in health care is not a trivial issue. It can and often does lead to death. This is especially egregious when the disease is curable. I was personally affected by this recently when my former sister-in-law refused treatment for curable breast cancer and instead followed an "alternative" pathway with nutrition, etc. When the cancer recurred, it was no longer curable, and she died a painful and unnecessary death. This behavior is inexplicable to me and very painful. I lost children with curable cancers when their parents sought such "alternative" care. Because of such awful situations, I am more comfortable if I can be trusted enough to provide treatment known to be effective and help minimize the harm that can come from unproven therapies.

The current political situation, which I will not belabor, is a more serious indication of growing confusion between fact and fiction, sometimes truth vs lies. This has adversely affected medical care, but it is not a new issue.

Finally, the principle of doing for others what you would accept for yourself is challenging, but provides, at least in my experience, an overarching guideline for the optimum practice of medicine. Thus, from the point of view of a religiously aware Jew, the practice of medicine should be sacred. I am sure that I have deviated often from this ideal professional behavior, but I also know that I have always tried to follow the right path and often succeeded. I am dismayed by what I see currently as a decreasing sense among medical professionals of the sacredness of their profession and a lack of a spiritual component in the care they provide. Certainly, this cannot be a good thing.

CHAPTER 22

This Is for the Birds
My Interest in Birding and How It Affected
My Medical Career and Life

When I first took up birding, courtesy of my friendship with Dr. Michael Linshaw of blessed memory, I was also just beginning to provide care for children with cancer. This took place at the Children's Hospital in Denver, Colorado where I was mentored by Dr. Charlene Holton who was trained at St. Jude's Hospital and was one of the first committed pediatric oncologists. These were challenging days in this burgeoning profession when nearly all of our patients died, and because, despite our good intentions, we had very few tools with which to reduce their suffering or prolong their lives. We were not a bunch of robots, so we suffered with our patients and their families. We survived and persisted because we took care of each other. We had a weekly conference with a psychologist to help us, not our patients, just to keep us going.

So, I guess you can understand how a person like me, who was dealing daily with suffering and death, might develop a passion for birds which in many ways served as a therapeutic diversion from my profession as well as my responsibilities as husband and father of young children. There was no downside to birding other than the challenge of finding time to do it, something that has not changed to this day. Birding affirms life, beauty, the harmony of nature, provides temporary relief from stress and worry, the joy of observing creatures that can overcome gravity in flight, all of these things the antithesis of what I faced the rest of the time.

Of course, things changed and we began to achieve both cures and reduction of suffering. With that came a dramatic increase in the pressure from parents and society to optimize each patient's chances for a good outcome. Later, when I switched from children to adults with brain tumors, this pressure lessened somewhat, but the losses were often worse because of the adult relationships that had developed. We had some success, but life was never easy, and there were many times when I didn't know how I could return to work the next day.

I have been asked literally dozens of times by friends, family, and the patients themselves why and how I do what I do. It's a reasonable question to ask because most people wouldn't do it. This includes most health care professionals. I'm not sure that I know the answer any more than I know why I am a birder except to say that it has something to do with a need to be "useful" and, perhaps, to understand life a little better in the process.

The term "useful" is part of this book's title and is borrowed from the novel The Cider House Rules by John Irving, one of my favorites which I have read several times. In that novel, Dr. Wilbur Larch, played by actor Michael Caine in the movie version, does abortions and cares for orphans with the same understated explanation, "to be of use". Part of Dr. Larch's tragedy was that he had little else in his life. Perhaps I understood this calamity subliminally when I got into birding. I also took up running, writing poetry, painting, music, backpacking, and writing these books for the same reason, to offset the frequently unacceptable outcomes of my patients and my work.

Having said all of the above, nothing has ever been sufficient to completely compensate for the stress of my calling as a cancer doctor. Whereas I am certainly not an accomplished birder, despite a wealth of adventures and successes, I can say that I have been an exceptional advocate for my patients, something that has delayed my retirement and made the process of "retirement" more painful. The writing of this book, which I have thoroughly enjoyed, has helped me through this process just as birding helped sustain my career. I hope this chapter, at least in part, explains and informs the rest of the story told in this book just as the writing process has helped me to better understand my own life, not just as a birder. I hope it has done the same for you.

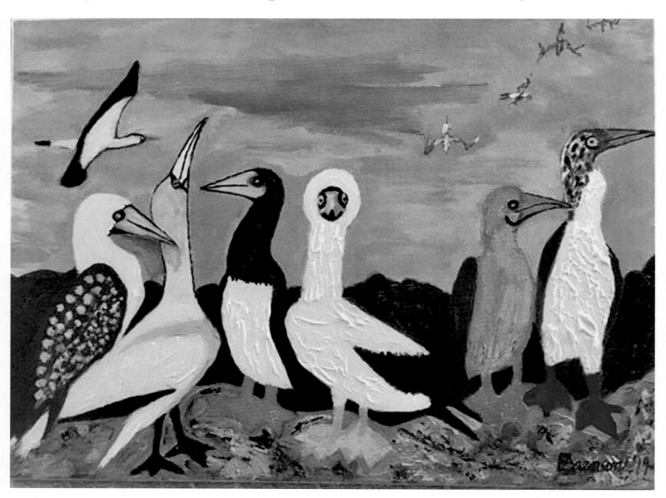

PAINTING BY THE AUTHOR

CHAPTER 23

Dayenu, Our Escape to Canada and Retirement

As the year 2020 began, my vision was no longer 20/20, and getting weaker as I approached my 75th birthday. Otherwise things seemed normal or normally abnormal as we began the fourth, and mercifully last, year of the Trump administration and last year that I would be practicing medicine. I watched dumbfounded as the United States Congress failed to remove this villain from office in the face of overwhelming evidence of corruption beyond anything seen before, at least in my lifetime. For me, it simply reinforced what I had been planning since the early 80s, that I needed to have a place to live in Canada and possibly to emigrate.

It all began when I visited Calgary, Alberta in 1981 to look at jobs as a pediatric hematologist-oncologist. I fell in love with the laid back and ostensibly more grounded life in Canada. I did not get the position, but I never stopped thinking about it. Of course, these were the days of Ronald Reagan, who was affable enough, but in my book an awful President. I had been active in the Civil Rights Movement and the anti-Viet Nam War movement even though I served two years in the Army Medical Corps. Frankly, I had never recovered from losing my political innocence when JFK was assassinated as I was walking to the dorms from the indoor rowing facility during my first year at Cornell University.

Now, with Donald Trump as President, it made Reagan look like a hero, which he was certainly not. The fact that nearly half of the American voters supported Trump and continue to support him made me feel like the USA had become for me, a Jew, the equivalent of Biblical Egypt, *mitzrayim,* the Hebrew word for dire straights, (not the rock band).

A few years back, my wife and I had travelled to Cape Breton in Nova Scotia and fell in love with its beauty and culture. We became acquainted with a realtor in the town of St. Peters, Sherry MacLeod, who, to say the least, is a real character. She lubricated us with local Scotch whiskey before taking us to see properties. We returned annually for the Celtic Colours Music Festival each October, and each time we looked at more properties. Finally, in 2018, we found the right one which I was fortunate enough to show to two of my high school classmates, Bruce Trumm and Kathleen Fulton, who had agreed to meet in Cape Breton for our annual reunion. They loved it as did we, and we bit. We closed on the property and took possession in August, 2019 after selling our larger loft in Denver. We kept the small unit next door since we could only spend 6 months per year in Canada, and I had not yet shut down my practice and career. Then came 2020.

I booked round trip tickets for my wife and me to go to our home in Cape Breton departing June 3rd, and returning November 1st. By the time of departure, I would be fully retired after nearly five decades as a physician which I have described in great detail in other chapters. I would see that all my patients were well situated with other providers and actively assist those few that were in need of acute care for as long as possible.

In February, we decided to make a trip to Cape Breton to check its winter condition and comfort and look into upgrading the heating system to something more modern and efficient than the oil burning furnace as well as something to provide cooling and dehumidification in the hotter summer months. We discovered that a heat pump(s) would take care of both and made the arrangements for installation. This gizmo stores heat from the environment and uses it as a source of energy to heat or cool as needed and also to remove humidity as desired. We were told that if we attended a home show in April, we would get a sizable discount, so we began planning another trip in April. Little did we know that our orderly plans would be disrupted and turned into chaos by the now infamous Covid19 pandemic which is rampant as I write this chapter.

At the time of our return to Denver in early February, we had begun seeing reports of an outbreak of a novel respiratory virus infection in Wuhan Province, China which was thought to have been transmitted to humans by bats and another animal like an armadillo which had been infected by the bats in outdoor markets. I remember attending an educational session at my synagogue about this time where I was asked by an old friend if she, who is a diabetic, should be worried about this virus. A few years ago, I told her not to be afraid of the avian flu, because I felt that it would burn itself out by destroying its susceptible avian hosts. I was right, and that virus faded away with minimal consequence. In this case, I told her that it appeared that the new coronavirus was extremely contagious from human to human as well as non-influenzal and, therefore, could infect many more people who had virtually no immunity to it. I had not considered how poorly a pandemic with a novel virus would be managed by the U.S. Government.

Unfortunately, I was correct, although the government apparently disagreed, and within days it was obvious that this was something unlike anything we had experienced in our lifetime. It brought to mind the plagues suffered by the Egyptian people which ultimately led to the Exodus. I rescheduled my flight to Canada from June to early April thinking that I would be safe that long and could leave on my own terms. I informed my company of my plans for early retirement so that there would be plenty of time to make arrangements to fill in for me.

As I accelerated my plan to make arrangements for my patients, I monitored the evolving pandemic and the egregious mismanagement thereof by the U.S. government (President). I also took into consideration my respiratory vulnerability and recent pneumonia which I probably got from being exposed to ultrasonic mist which I was using for one of my wound care patients. It quickly became obvious, and I was told so by my doctors, that I should not be working in a health care facility and should retire, or at least work from a distance, immediately. It also became apparent that I was at risk of being unable to cross the border into Canada as travel restrictions went into effect. Thus, within a span of 48 hours, thank god, I resolved to end my medical career much more abruptly than I wanted, and literally flee for the border where we would not need to cross the Red Sea, but would face a Canadian Customs officer instead. A plane was not an option, so we decided to drive.

I made this decision on Friday, March 13, and my wife insisted that we depart early in the morning of March 15, thank god, headed for the Canadian border-crossing into Manitoba called Pembina which is one hour north of Grand Forks, North Dakota. We scrambled to get ready and make sure we had enough food to avoid going into stores or restaurants and took a few extra things that we could take because we were driving. We left Denver in the dark at 5 a.m. on Sunday, March 15, and arrived in Grand Forks at 8 p.m. having lost one hour to Central Time. We stayed in a Hilton on the campus of U. North Dakota where we passed the huge hockey pavilion appropriate for U.N.D.'s perennial collegiate hockey power, probably the largest building in town. The drive had been scenic, and we saw a great deal of wildlife, especially huge flocks of snow geese, which all seemed reassuring, but we worried in silence about our border-crossing the next morning.

As we prepared for our trip, we had an early morning telephone conference with our Canadian immigration attorney, Ms. Jamie Taylor, who told us that we might be held up at the border and to be sure to have plenty of documentation of our commitment to being American citizens and to downplay our interest in Canada other than as part- time visitors with our own property as our destination. This conversation was useful, but also created a vicarious *déjà vu* of escape from the Nazis as memorialized in The Sound of Music; our anxiety level escalated.

We arose early to head for the border, but our progress was slowed first by a snale freight train that blocked the tracks for 30 minutes, then by drifting snow from a snowstorm that passed through during the night. We arrived at Customs at about 9 a.m. at which time we hoped to encounter an agent who was fresh and not yet stressed from the day. We had no idea how we would be received. It was a young lady, very businesslike, very dry, who asked where we were going, how long we planned to stay, and if we had any symptoms of acute illness. She was satisfied with our honest answers, including why we were driving so far, checked our passports, and let us go. We drove slowly forward to savor the moment, looked at each other, smiled, fist-pumped, and proceeded *en route* to Thunder Bay on the north shore of Lake Superior.

To say that this was a great relief does not do justice to this moment. We were nearly paralyzed with dread, but neither showed it to the other. Now we were in Canada where we at least felt safer and could make it to our isolated sanctuary in Cape Breton and stay there as long as we wanted as long as we played by the rules. By that afternoon, several of our friends informed us of the imminent closing of the border, and by the next day, it was closed to U.S. citizens except special cases. Maybe it was luck, maybe it was good instincts, maybe it was something else. Doesn't matter; we made it, thank god.

As we headed for Thunder Bay, I envisioned a romantic seaport town with gorgeous views of Lake Superior, *gichi gami*, which Aura had never seen, but where I had gone to summer camp as a pre-teen and along which I had run the Grandma's Marathon.

As we descended from the woods into town, there was no view and everything looked past its prime. That included our inn which tried to charge us for two days when we only stayed one. My hopes of finding a place to eat some fresh Lake Superior fish were unfulfilled, and we left the next morning headed for Timmins, Ontario instead of Sault St. Marie in order to stay farther north and avoid the larger cities of Toronto and Montreal.

We picked up our breakfasts in a bag, which was the only kind of breakfast we would get on our journey, and headed for Timmins with a full tank of gas, thank god. We traveled more than two hundred very scenic miles before we found a place to get gas or use the bathroom. This led to several instances of stopping by large mounds of plowed snow, well above my head, opening both doors on the snow side of the car, and relieving myself as cars and trucks passed by. My limited bladder capacity is now measured by the distance between spots of yellowed snow. The scenery was spectacular, deep snow, a few snowmobilers, spruce and birch trees, and innumerable small flocks of various finches which seemed to be getting something they needed from the snowbanks along the highway.

As we drove through what is truly the great white north, it struck me how treacherous this route would be in foul weather of which we had none, thank god. We arrived safely at our destination in early evening, our third full day of driving. In the morning we experienced once again the surreal sight of our breakfasts in bags on a table in what would normally would have been the restaurant. There was a pleasant and apologetic employee nearby who kept her distance, but told us that there were other things available if we weren't satisfied with a muffin, apple, yogurt, and boxed juice. We were satisfied, served ourselves some coffee and headed for our next stop, Mont-Laurier, Quebec.

The only thing noteworthy about this day's drive was our entry into rural French-speaking Quebec. We arrived comparatively early and offered some French to the clerk who was separated from us by a large table and glass barrier. Her boss paced as we checked in and were told that we should enter our room from the outside door and could order food from the adjoining bistro. It was obvious that Canada was in full pandemic mode, something that I had not anticipated, but undoubtably a good thing. Despite the early hour, we fell asleep almost immediately after downing our meal of chicken fingers and limp French fries. Our next drive would be a long one, but one which would get us into southern New Brunswick where we would be within reach the next day of our destination and home, thank god. We had started collecting food and drinks at each stop in order to make sure that we would not starve once we arrived in Cape Breton.

The ten- hour drive to Fredericton, New Brunswick took us north of Montreal and across the St. Lawrence Seaway at Trois Rivieres to avoid Quebec City against the wishes of our GPS. This put us on highway 20 which takes a circuitous route around the northern part of Maine in order to enter New Brunswick without crossing the U.S. border, something that was no longer an option. I would estimate that this route took us an extra two hours. As we headed south along the Maine/ New Brunswick border, we saw numerous signs warning us to be on the alert for moose in the road. A high- speed collision in a car with a moose in likely to be fatal for both the animal and the occupants of the vehicle, so we were vigilant. The trick is to avoid driving at night which we accomplished, thank god, and arrived unscathed after another long drive in Fredericton, a very picturesque town along the St. Johns River. We stayed in the Bonvoy Delta hotel where we also had stayed the previous August.

The excellent restaurant was closed, and no one came closer than six feet as mandated. The difference was a shocking reminder of the gravity of the situation we were all in. We slept well and departed promptly at 7 a.m. with our bagged breakfasts and our thumping hearts on the last leg to McNabs Cove, Cape Breton where we arrived, safe and possibly sound, by mid- afternoon, 3500 miles, six days, and 44 hours of driving from Denver, on March 20, 2020, the year of the great Covid19 pandemic, happy to be where we were, and with no idea when we would leave Cape Breton or see our families and friends again in person. Within hours we found chicken soup and other goodies on our doorstep, left there by our unseen friend, Sherry MacLeod, who is one of the compelling reasons why we chose Cape Breton, thank god, as our sanctuary before we had the remotest notion what a true sanctuary it would come to be. We appreciated the rapid and coordinated response of the Canadian government which inconvenienced, but protected us.

As I wrote what you just read, and inspired by my daughter Patty who is always an inspiration, I began to realize that our personal journey was surprisingly similar to famous epic journeys in history and literature, especially the Exodus of the Hebrews from Egypt which will be celebrated in a Passover *seder*, (a ceremony conducted in a specific order,) in a few weeks as it has been for millenia. In this ceremony, which must be virtual this year under the pandemic constraints, it is traditional to repeat with gratitude the many "acts of god" without which things certainly would have turned out differently. After each act, we say "Dayenu" which means it would have been enough, and for us, we say "dayenu", for whatever it was that brought us through our own epic journey unscathed and for which we will always by humbled and grateful.

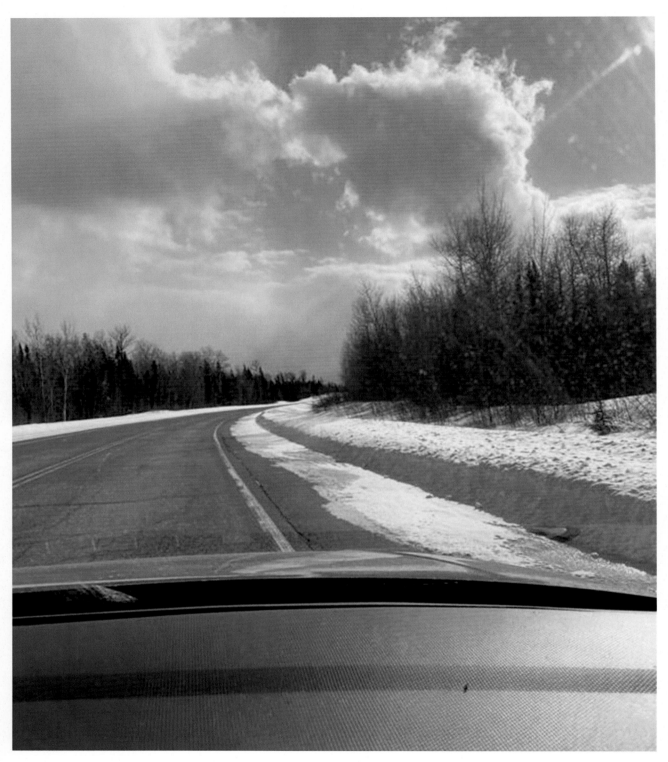

WE CROSS THE GREAT WHITE NORTH
INTO RETIREMENT IN CAPE BRETON

CONCLUSION

In these twenty-three chapters I have told the true story of my nearly five decades in the medical profession as a cancer and blood doctor as well as a specialist in wound care and hyperbaric oxygen medicine. This story is an intimate and personal one as well as a history of the many major events in medicine that I experienced along the way. Having told this saga, I have taken time to give tribute to a select group of those fellow medical professionals and teachers whose work and lives have had the greatest impact. I have also taken the opportunity to ventilate some of my concerns and frustrations as I look back on a long career and look forward to retirement (or some variation thereof short of the ultimate retirement). I have explained my reasons for optimism in the face of the current daunting challenges faced by my beloved profession.

The writing of this book has given me the pleasure of reliving in detail a rich and relentlessly informative life in medicine. As I did so, I became increasingly convinced that I had learned some things from which others might benefit or at least see things from a different perspective. If I am correct in this belief, I will be honored to have provided this. If not, I won't regret for one second my career itself or the pleasure of putting it all into words. As for the title, TO BE of USE, I make no claim of altruism; if one can be of use in any capacity, especially for the benefit of others, one might shamelessly welcome respect or even love in return. I do not believe this prospect diminishes the achievement in any way; it is simply the way the world works, when it works.

Edward Arenson MD CWSP, January, 2020

Printed in the United States
By Bookmasters